KETO FOR VEGETARIANS

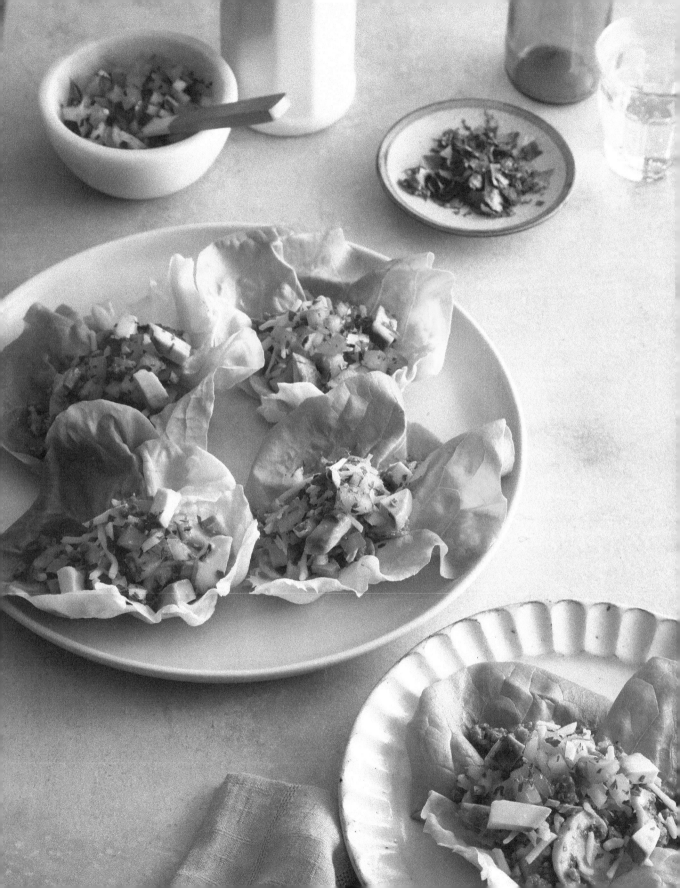

KETO FOR VEGETARIANS

Lose Weight and Improve Health on a Plant-Based Ketogenic Diet

LISA DANIELSON

Photography by Laura Flippen

ROCKRIDGE PRESS

For general information on our other products and services or to obtain technical support, please contact our Customer Care Department within the United States at (866) 744-2665, or outside the United States at (510) 253-0500.

Rockridge Press publishes its books in a variety of electronic and print formats. Some content that appears in print may not be available in electronic books, and vice versa.

Interior and Cover Designer: Michael Cook
Art Producer: Karen Williams
Editor: Justin Hartung
Production Editor: Jenna Dutton

Photography © 2020 Laura Flippen. Food styling by Cole Church.

Author photo courtesy of © Maggie Yahvah Photography.

Cover: Creamed Spinach with Eggs. Photography by: Laura Flippen

ISBN: Print 978-1-64152-550-3 | eBook 978-1-64152-551-0

R0

To all the people out there taking charge of their health one vegetable at a time.

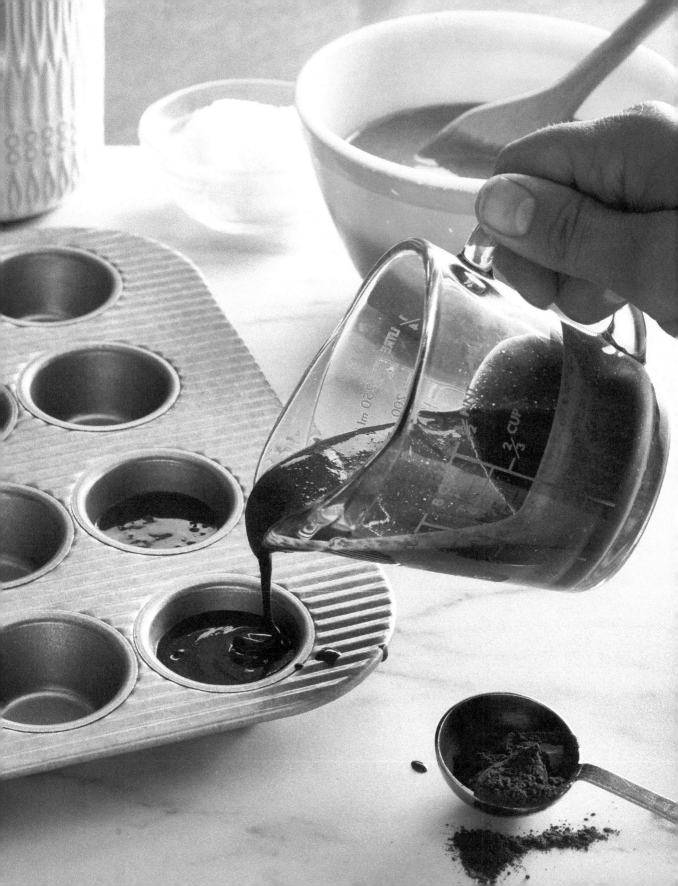

CONTENTS

Introduction viii

CHAPTER ONE   Vegetarian Keto Basics *1*

CHAPTER TWO   Getting Started *7*

CHAPTER THREE   14-Day Meal Plan and Beyond *17*

CHAPTER FOUR   Breakfast and Smoothies *31*

CHAPTER FIVE   Salads, Soups, and Sandwiches *51*

CHAPTER SIX   Snacks, Appetizers, and Savory Fat Bombs *73*

CHAPTER SEVEN   Hearty Main Dishes *95*

CHAPTER EIGHT   Desserts *115*

CHAPTER NINE   Staples, Sauces, and Dressings *137*

Measurement Conversions 148
Resources 149
Index 150

INTRODUCTION ·

For the past few years, the ketogenic diet has been all the rage. As a nutritionist, I hear questions all the time about what exactly this diet is. Some wonder if it is simply a new version of the Atkins diet, or perhaps the popular low-carb diet that was around in the early 1990s. It is neither of those, but it is another tool for people to lose weight, feel better, and have more energy. Most keto diets feature meat as the main component of each meal. And that is fine for people who eat meat. But what if you want to try a ketogenic diet and you don't eat meat, or you've decided to stop eating meat? This book is for you. Because the recipes focus mainly on fat with a side of protein, meat becomes unnecessary.

I have roughly 31 years of a vegetarian lifestyle under my belt. At a young age, I knew meat wasn't for me. Naturally, my mom thought it was just a phase, but after a few years, it became more of a reality. Our meat-and-potatoes family had a little less meat here and there, and ordering out at burger joints became difficult (this was the mid-eighties and veggie burgers were nonexistent). In my early twenties, I met the man of my dreams and settled into married life. During the course of my first pregnancy I gained 80 pounds, and even though I gave birth to a beautiful eight-pound baby boy, I had quite a bit of weight to lose. I learned that complete nutrition for a vegetarian was a bit different from what I had previously thought. Over the next two years, I lost 60 pounds. Sixteen years (and three more babies) later, I have maintained that weight loss while still enjoying the foods I love and without having to eat meat.

Because I am a weight-loss coach, the ketogenic diet intrigued me. The science behind it is compelling, as was watching the transformation of my clients. Four to six weeks into their keto diets, I would hear the same thing: "I'm sick of eating so much meat." Traditional keto uses the fattiest meats—beef, bacon, sausage, etc.—in order to hit those fat macros. But those meats tend to be the ones that some people don't enjoy as much as they enjoy chicken or turkey; therefore, their meals got boring . . . really fast. I needed to help find them more keto options with less meat.

There are many healthy vegetarian fat sources available that can be added to any plant-based meal. Avocado, seeds, coconut, olive oil, cheese, and nuts are all solid options. Our bodies are much more adaptable to plant-based fats than animal fats. We are able to process them more quickly and more efficiently, allowing for maximum blood flow, which aids in our recovery, endurance, and overall health.

Being a vegetarian isn't without its challenges. Options when eating out can be limited, but the good news is that most restaurants realize that not everyone wants to eat meat at every single meal. Interestingly, most of my female clients say that they would be happy never eating meat again.

Is this diet right for you? People who struggle with inflammation, autoimmune diseases, or adrenal fatigue have experienced wonderful benefits from eating a vegetarian ketogenic diet, as have those who simply want to lose weight, have more energy, and see fast results. Making the change to this diet will take some work in the beginning, but I promise you, the end goal is worth it! I applaud you for taking the time to listen to your body and for making bold decisions about your nutrition.

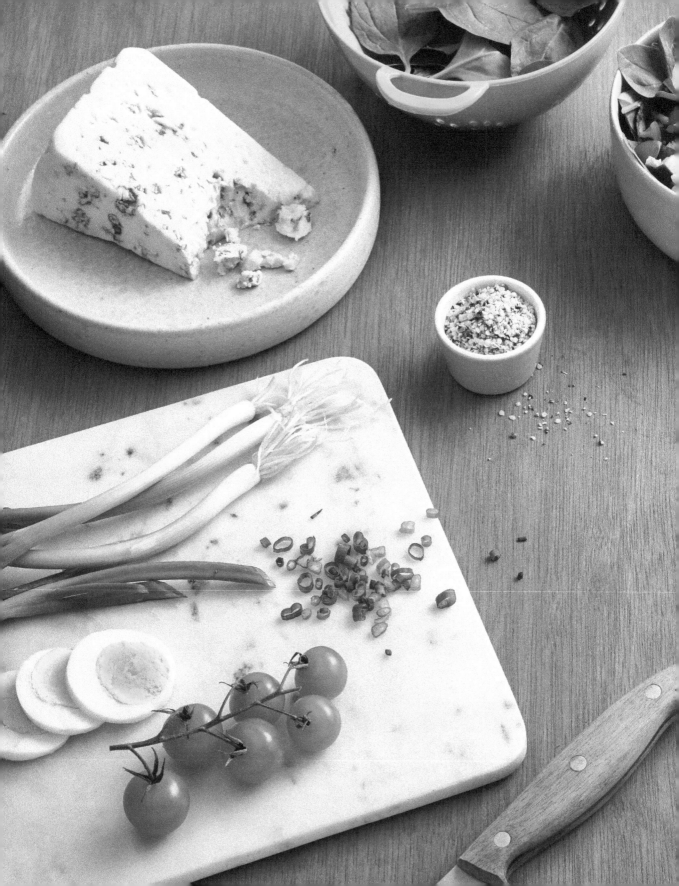

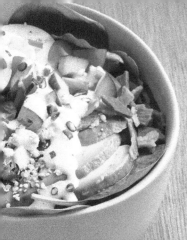

CHAPTER ONE

Vegetarian Keto Basics

If you're holding this book in your hands, you've likely already heard about the ketogenic diet, which has reached new heights of popularity in recent years. You've probably also heard about how the classic version of this diet entails eating large amounts of meat. So, you might have been wondering if there's a version of the keto diet that will work for vegetarians. Good news: You can enjoy all the benefits of the diet and still eat vegetarian—no meat necessary. This book will show you how. In this first chapter, you'll get an overview of the ketogenic diet, you'll learn about macros and the importance of counting them in order to stay in ketosis (more about that later), and you'll understand how to become keto-adapted as a vegetarian eater. You'll also learn more about the diet's many benefits, including its anti-inflammatory properties. Most people are eager to jump straight into cooking the recipes, but it's very important that you understand the basic keto principles before diving in. The information you're about to read may seem a little complicated at first, but don't worry: You'll soon get the hang of it and be on your way to a veggie-filled keto life in no time.

Ketogenic Diet 101

You might be surprised to learn that the ketogenic diet has been around a long time—about 100 years, in fact. It was initially developed to help children who were experiencing seizures.

But what exactly is keto? The basic premise of the ketogenic diet is to eat low carb and high fat. This is counterintuitive to many of us who have traditionally been taught that fat is bad for us and we should certainly not eat much of it if we hope to lose weight. The truth is, though, that by eating enough of the correct types of fat, your body will enter a metabolic state known as "nutritional ketosis." It might seem more than a little crazy to think you can lose fat by eating fat, but the scientific basis is sound. Our bodies mainly run on glucose, which is the product of the breakdown of carbohydrates such as rice, grains, pasta, cereals, etc. But when we drastically reduce our carbohydrate intake and add a high amount of fat to our diet, our bodies switch from using carbohydrates as fuel to using fat as fuel, and we are then able to reach ketosis.

Nutritional ketosis allows your body to become a fat-burning machine by turning fat into ketones in the liver. Ketones are a secondary form of energy that our bodies need in order to function. This backup fuel system allows us to trick our metabolism into burning stored fat rather than carbohydrates. These ketones become the primary source of energy for our organs, muscles, and brain to function properly. Many researchers believe that ketones are a more efficient fuel source than carbohydrates because they burn more slowly, giving your body a more sustaining source of energy.

How Can It Help You?

The ketogenic diet is immensely popular thanks to its wide array of benefits. Various studies show the diet can reduce inflammation, increase energy, decrease food cravings (especially for sugar), help clear skin, improve fat burning, slow the effects of aging, and lower the risk of chronic disease. However, one of the most talked-about advantages to living a keto lifestyle is mental clarity.

Neurological inflammation has been linked to poor cognitive function, as well as depression and anxiety. Just about everyone who has followed the ketogenic diet claims to have experienced the benefit of clearer thinking. Neurological inflammation is most likely caused by an overall inflammation that in turn affects the brain by increasing focal brain inflammation.

As mentioned previously, keto was initially used to treat children with epilepsy. Since then, it has proved effective in battling serious illnesses such as diabetes,

Parkinson's, and autoimmune diseases, including Hashimoto's. The diet has been shown to increase glutathione, a combination of amino acids that's your body's most powerful detoxifier (and something often found lacking in people with autoimmune issues). While in nutritional ketosis, your body will naturally produce more glutathione, which acts as a powerful antioxidant that reduces oxidative stress caused by a poor diet, stress, or infection.

Weight loss is also a result of eating a ketogenic diet, and it often happens quickly. Fundamentally, when you starve your body of carbs and sugar, your blood sugar decreases. Your body responds by switching to the alternate form of energy—ketones—and then for as long as you stay in ketosis, your body will continue to burn fat. It is not uncommon for people to lose most of their unwanted pounds in the early stages of keto, while others experience a steady weight loss for as long as they are in ketosis.

Understanding Macros

Macros, which is short for *macronutrients*, refers to the three main nutrients our bodies need to function: protein, fats, and carbohydrates. Your body converts these nutrients into energy for your brain, muscles, and organs. In most diets, macros are tailored toward a person's body type, activity level, and nutritional needs. For example, some diets recommend a 30 percent fat, 35 percent protein, and 35 percent carbohydrate split of daily calories. Vegetarian ketogenic macros, on the other hand, typically target 70 percent fat, 20 percent protein, and 10 percent net carbs, most of those carbs coming from vegetables.

You may have seen the terms "total carbs" and "net carbs" on food labels. "Total carbs" is the tally of all the sugars, fiber, and indigestible starch in a food item. Our bodies need fiber in order to be able to excrete waste products efficiently, but because we cannot digest fiber, it has no effect on blood sugar levels. "Net carbs" refers to the carbohydrates that can be converted into sugar in our bodies and therefore affect blood sugar levels.

When calculating net carbs, it's important to ignore sugar alcohols. These are organic compounds found in vegetables, fruit, and many sugar-free products. They have a much lower impact on blood sugar than regular sugars, which is why they are typically subtracted when calculating net carbs. Here's the formula:

Total carbohydrates - fiber - sugar alcohols = net carbs

While you are on the ketogenic diet, you will want to pay attention to the foods you buy to make sure you keep within the 10 percent carbohydrate ratio for your total overall daily calories. The good news is that you don't need to carry around a calculator to track your macros on the keto diet. There are several helpful apps (available for a small monthly fee) that you can customize for individual macro percentages. Some of my favorites are MyFitnessPal, CalorieKing, and Carb Manager. You may also find it helpful to keep a food journal, at least until you become accustomed to the diet.

Benefits and Challenges of a Vegetarian Keto Diet

As previously mentioned, many people associate the keto diet with having to consume a great deal of meat, particularly fatty steak and bacon. Not enough studies have been done to calculate the health risks of such high meat consumption on a long-term basis. Even if you're not a vegetarian, you may have come to this book because you're curious about the ketogenic diet and eager to try it for its multiple benefits, but you are concerned about the diet's overreliance on meat consumption. The good news is that a vegetarian keto diet is absolutely possible and comes with its own set of benefits.

Most vegetarians rely heavily on carbohydrates such as beans, rice, pasta, and bread to keep them full. One challenge of following the ketogenic vegetarian diet, therefore, is figuring out how to replace those carbs with a higher amount of fat and protein. Fortunately, if you're already a plant-based eater, you're likely used to alternative forms of protein such as edamame, tofu, eggs, and some dairy products. Switching from using carbs for fuel to using fat should be fairly easy for you since you are already comfortable with making substitutions.

People decide to adopt a ketogenic diet for different reasons, whether it is to manage their blood sugar better, to lose weight, or even to reduce dependence on certain prescription medications. All of these benefits can come from eating keto. Plant-based diets have some pretty incredible benefits as well, including lowering high blood pressure, keeping cholesterol in check, and reducing overall inflammation that can be caused by animal proteins. So, it only makes sense to combine the vegetarian and ketogenic diets into one super diet.

Ketosis and Becoming Keto-Adapted

Another term associated with the ketogenic diet is "keto-adapted," also known as "being in ketosis" or "fat-adapted." The term refers to the metabolic state in which your body's primary fuel source has switched from glucose (carbs) to ketones. Essentially, this means your body is now burning stored fat for energy.

You'll use the ketogenic diet to get into ketosis by eating fewer carbs and less protein, eating more fat, listening to your body, and getting more sleep. But how do you know when you have become keto-adapted?

When you suspect you are in ketosis, you need to measure the ketones in your body. There are three primary ways to test your ketone levels: a blood ketone meter (small finger prick), breath testing, and urine keto strips. Some studies show that using a blood ketone meter is the most accurate method; these are readily available online, but they can be expensive. A cheaper, noninvasive option is breath testing, which measures acetone levels in your breath. Urine keto strips are considered the most inaccurate of the three, but if you are only wanting to test during the beginning phases of keto, these are a viable option and can be found at your local pharmacy.

So, using one of these three methods, how do you know that you are in ketosis? With blood testing, anything above 0.5 millimoles indicates ketosis. With breath testing, the detection of acetone means you are in ketosis. Finally, with urine strips, there will be a color change: Dark purple usually means there are ketones present (just make sure to follow the chart on the side of the bottle).

In the next chapter, you'll learn the steps to becoming keto-adapted with a long-term plan tailored just for you.

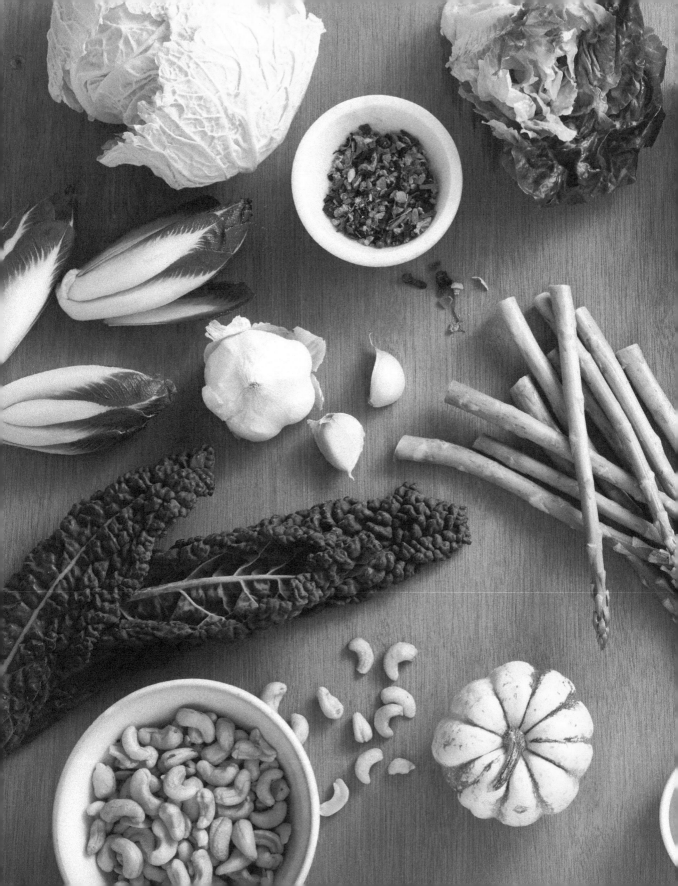

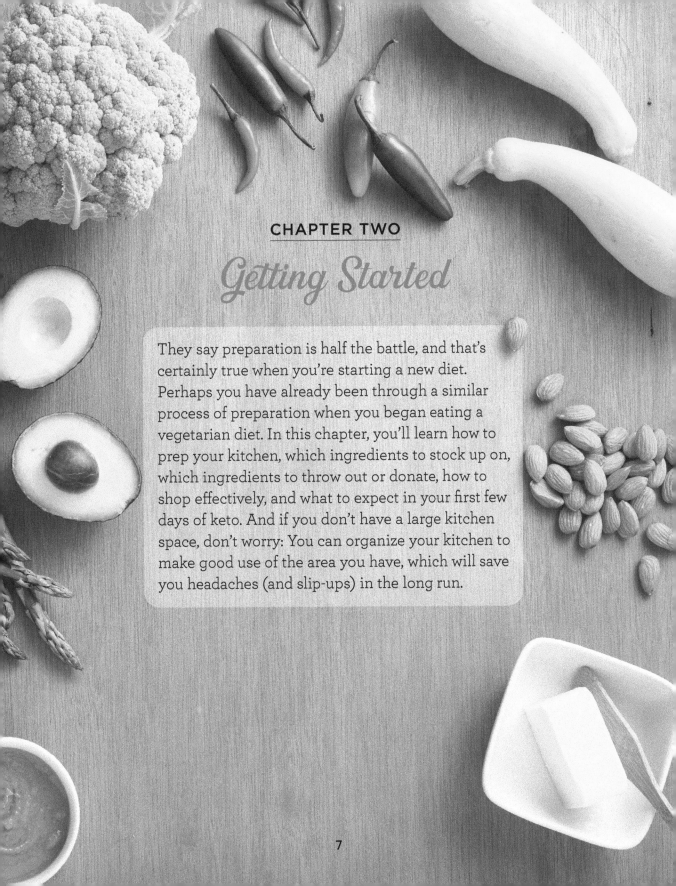

CHAPTER TWO

Getting Started

They say preparation is half the battle, and that's certainly true when you're starting a new diet. Perhaps you have already been through a similar process of preparation when you began eating a vegetarian diet. In this chapter, you'll learn how to prep your kitchen, which ingredients to stock up on, which ingredients to throw out or donate, how to shop effectively, and what to expect in your first few days of keto. And if you don't have a large kitchen space, don't worry: You can organize your kitchen to make good use of the area you have, which will save you headaches (and slip-ups) in the long run.

Kitchen Prep

The first step is to figure out exactly what to remove from your kitchen and what to buy to get your vegetarian ketogenic pantry ready. In order to get you into ketosis as quickly as possible, you'll want to get rid of all the non-keto treats that can and will tempt you. I believe that as long as you have a good stockpile of the foods you need and can eat, you will be less likely to cheat and/or binge. For the purposes of this prep step, I am assuming that you are a vegetarian already, so I do not list meats in the foods to get rid of. If you currently eat meat, obviously any meats in your refrigerator or freezer will have to find a new home.

Stock Up On . . .

(* = eat in moderation):

- Almonds
- Arugula
- Asparagus
- Avocado
- Bell peppers
- Black coffee
- Blackberries*
- Blueberries*
- Broccoli
- Brussels sprouts
- Butter
- Cabbage
- Cashews
- Cauliflower
- Celery
- Cheese
- Chia seeds
- Chile peppers
- Cream cheese
- Cucumbers
- Eggs
- Flaxseeds
- Garlic
- Heavy cream
- Herbal teas
- Kale
- Lettuce, all types
- Macadamia nuts
- Mushrooms
- Nut butters (natural)
- Olives
- Onions*
- Pecans
- Pickles
- Pumpkin
- Pumpkin seeds
- Raspberries*
- Sauerkraut
- Scallions
- Spaghetti squash
- Spinach
- Strawberries*
- Sunflower seeds
- Tomatoes*
- Walnuts
- Water, plain and sparkling
- Yellow squash
- Zucchini

Get Rid of . . .

all starchy vegetables

- Carrots
- Corn
- Potatoes
- Sweet potatoes

carb-heavy fruits

- Apples
- Bananas
- Mangos
- Oranges
- Pineapples

other carb-heavy foods

- Barley
- Beans, all types
- Cereals
- Chips

- Crackers
- Legumes
- Millet
- Oats
- Pasta
- Quinoa
- Rice
- Sprouted grains
- Wheat

sugary foods
- Agave
- Cane sugar
- Donuts
- Dried fruits
- Fructose corn syrup
- Honey
- Ice cream

- Juices
- Peas
- Raw sugar
- Sodas
- Sugar-added yogurts
- Turbnado sugar

Lose the Booze?

Often, the first question many keto newbies ask is whether they can still drink alcohol. Unfortunately, there isn't a straightforward answer. An important point to consider is that your tolerance for alcohol is much lower during ketosis.

Additionally, alcoholic drinks, even the low-carb varieties, contain carbohydrates, and you'll want to save your carb allowance for nutrient-dense foods such as vegetables. You can still drink alcohol and stay in ketosis, but because it is a carb, it is the first thing your liver will process, which means you would be putting a hold on the fat-burning process until your body finishes metabolizing the alcohol. Drinking alcohol can therefore really slow down your fat loss. The entire goal of keto is to deplete your glycogen stores so your body burns fat instead of glucose, so adding alcohol on a low-carbohydrate diet is counterintuitive.

Later in your keto journey, you may decide to indulge a little bit. Your best choices for alcohol while on keto are the hard liquors such as tequila, vodka, dry wine, or whiskey. These drinks are just a combination of alcohol and water, which won't affect your insulin levels in the way that other sugar-loaded alcoholic beverages will. A good rule of thumb is to remember that clear alcoholic drinks are more keto-friendly.

Alternatives to Vegetarian Staples

Bad habits can be hard to break, as you may already know from previous, perhaps unsuccessful, attempts. But with just a bit of time and dedication, bad habits can be changed to better habits. The trick is to find better alternatives. Of course, it would be lovely if you could continue to eat everything you habitually eat (think pizza, burgers, and ice cream) and still get into and maintain ketosis, but that just isn't going to happen. So, when those cravings hit, you need some healthy alternatives you can enjoy.

- Carb-heavy fruits (see the table on page 8) are out of the question while on keto. Some better options are any and all types of berries, such as blueberries, boysenberries, raspberries, and blackberries. Other fruits that can be added include avocados, prickly pears, olives (any color and kind), and coconut.
- Potatoes are a staple in the standard American diet but don't work well when trying to get into ketosis. If you find yourself longing for a big bowl of mashed potatoes with butter, keep the butter and simply replace the potatoes with mashed cauliflower.
- Traditional bread is also a no-no, but the keto world has a wonderful replacement called keto bread (see page 143). It is thick and hearty and makes terrific sandwiches, as you will discover if you try the Ultimate Grilled Cheese (page 66).
- Pasta for keto typically will be made from a vegetable. Spiralized zucchini and yellow squash mimic the texture of pasta but contain far fewer carbs.
- Pizza is still an option on keto, except you will replace the wheat crust with a psyllium husk crust. And remember you can load up on the cheese, which is arguably the tastiest part anyway.
- Beans are too carb-heavy for keto, so for the most part they are off-limits. However, two foods from the legume family that do work for keto (in moderate portions) are black soybeans and green beans. Black soybeans contain only 1 gram of net carbs per 100-gram serving, and green beans contain 3.6 grams of net carbs per serving.

Special Keto Ingredients

To make ketosis easier to achieve and maintain, I recommend purchasing a few specialty items. Although these are not strictly necessary, they are certainly nice to have.

- **Sweeteners** to look for instead of regular granulated sugar are monk fruit, stevia, or Swerve.
- **Coconut and almond flour** are useful substitutes for white flour in baking and other keto dishes.
- **Organic virgin coconut oil** is a staple keto item; other recommended oils to use are extra-virgin olive oil, avocado oil, grapeseed oil, and, of course, butter.
- **Organic cocoa powder** can take the place of chocolate chips for keto cooking and baking, and I recommend also purchasing Lily's Dark Chocolate Baking Chips, which are sweetened with stevia.
- **MCT oil** is another keto basic. You can find this in actual oil form or powdered for convenience. BHB products are also good to have on hand. These are lab-created ketones that start the process of ketosis and thereby increase body metabolism.

- **Xanthan gum** can be easily found in the baking aisle of your local grocery store. This can be used to thicken sauces and soups.
- **Salt**, such as pink Himalayan or mined salt, will be extremely important when battling any symptoms of keto flu (see page 12) and for fueling your body properly by keeping it hydrated.
- **Electrolytes** are important to help avoid headaches, light-headedness, and fatigue.
- **Nuts**, for cooking and snacking, are great to keep on hand. They are portable, shelf-stable, and rich in fat. Try macadamia nuts, cashews, and almonds.

ESSENTIAL KITCHEN TOOLS

MUST HAVES

- 8-by-8-inch and 9-by-13-inch casserole dishes
- 9-inch pie plate
- Blender
- Bread pan
- Cutting board(s)
- Grater
- Hand mixer
- Kitchen knives
- Measuring spoons and cups
- Muffin tin
- Nonstick skillet
- Pizza cutter
- Saucepans
- Silicone fat bomb molds
- Spatulas
- Stockpot
- Strainer
- Vegetable peeler

NICE TO HAVES

- 2-ounce dressing cups with lids
- Electric ice cream maker
- Electric kettle
- Food processor
- Food scale
- Immersion blender
- Meal-prep containers
- Muffin tin
- Potato masher
- Pressure cooker
- Silicone baking sheets
- Slow cooker
- Spiralizer
- Stand mixer
- Waffle maker

Smart Shopping

Now that you have a good idea of the kitchen tools and equipment that will be helpful and the foods you need to stock up on, it's time to head to the grocery store.

Eating healthy doesn't necessarily have to be expensive, and you won't be buying any meat, which will help keep your bill lower, too. The pricier items will include cheese, nuts, oil, butter, and eggs, but you can shop at your favorite grocery store and stock up on many items during sales. When it comes to fresh produce, buying fruits and vegetables in season and using them to create your favorite dishes is a good way to keep costs down and flavors and nutrition up. Keeping meals simple will always lead to a smaller grocery bill and less time prepping in the kitchen.

There are some other ways to shop smart, too. The most important tip might be to never go grocery shopping when you are hungry (this will keep you from overspending). Always take a list of what you need for the week, and check off each item as you put it in your cart. Shop the outer aisles first, as that is where most stores place their fresh produce. Try reaching out to some friends to find out if any of them have been or are on keto and would be willing to tag along on your first grocery store run. They can be helpful in pointing out the foods to buy and the foods to avoid.

Tips for Success

Life can throw some major curveballs, as we know, and for some reason, they often show up at the beginning of a new diet, leading to the derailment of your best-laid plans, and tempting treats and snacks are suddenly everywhere you look. Getting into ketosis will take some effort and persistence, but the benefits you reap will make your dedication worthwhile. In this section, you will learn tips for success when it comes to potentially tricky situations such as managing the keto flu, fasting, and eating out. The more knowledge you arm yourself with at the beginning of your diet, the better your results will be and the more your confidence will grow.

Managing Keto Flu

Keto flu. What is it? It certainly doesn't sound good, but fortunately, if you happen to experience it, it doesn't last long. As you know, your body is accustomed to relying on glucose (carbohydrates) for energy; the keto diet forces it to use ketones for energy instead. If your customary diet has not been the healthiest, your body will be metabolically inflexible, and making the switch to keto will take a bit longer and be a bit harder. You might experience symptoms of the keto flu, which are sugar cravings, nausea, dizziness, brain fog, fatigue, or stomach irritability. These symptoms usually show up in the first week and can last for three to five days. Generally, they are caused by one to three things: low levels of electrolytes, desire for carbs, and difficulty switching from carbs to ketones.

The good news is you can help ease any symptoms until your body switches over to ketosis. The first thing to try is adding more salt to your diet. You can do this either by simply salting your food more liberally or by dissolving about 1 tablespoon of salt in water to create a "salt shot" drink. Make sure you are drinking plenty of water and electrolytes so you stay properly hydrated. Next, consider raising your calorie intake by around 100 and seeing if you notice a difference in your symptoms. Exercising, eating more fat, and also taking BHBs can help get you into ketosis faster, which in turn will alleviate any keto flu symptoms.

Intermittent Fasting

Intermittent fasting is a catchall term for a number of different eating/fasting schedules and has long been a helpful tool for people to see results and burn fat more quickly. The following are a few different options that you can consider:

Skipped meals: This technique involves skipping one meal a day to help induce ketosis. Most commonly, breakfast is skipped.

Eating windows: This method works by limiting the eating window to one eight-hour period—for example, between 11 a.m. and 7 p.m. The remaining hours are spent fasting.

24- or 48-hour cleanse: This is an extended period of fasting that helps speed up getting into ketosis.

I recommend trying a 24-hour cleanse during the first week of keto. You may find it easiest to do it at the beginning of the week, either Sunday or Monday. It's essential that you continue to drink liquids, such as water with lemon, herbal teas, electrolytes, powdered greens, MCT oil, apple cider vinegar, and black tea, to get you through the full 24 hours. I often suggest a noon-to-noon fast so it doesn't feel as though there is an entire day of not eating.

As you become keto-adapted, fasting will become easier and easier. Fasting is not required for keto; it is just another tool to help you reach your goals more quickly. The high amount of fat in your keto diet will keep you feeling satisfied for longer, and your body will be better at using your stored fat for fuel.

Meal Prep and Shortcuts

Prepping meals is one of the best tips for success with the keto diet. Knowing what you are going to eat next and having it ready and close at hand will reduce stress and eliminate last-minute food decisions that may not be the best choices. Cooking recipes in batches, dividing them into individual meals, and storing them in the refrigerator or freezer will help keep you on the right track to ketosis. Most of the recipes in this book will store well in the refrigerator for three to five days, which will give you endless meal options if you decided to meal prep your food. Setting yourself up ahead of time with suitable meal prep and storage containers will make doing this a breeze, and don't forget the sheer satisfaction of opening the refrigerator to see it full of food ready to go.

Another option, which is both convenient and budget-friendly, is to save leftovers from dinner and use them for lunch the next day. You can even get creative and use leftover veggies as an ingredient in an omelet, a sauce for pouring over a bed of zoodles, or soup. Don't feel limited to the recipes provided in this book; use your new knowledge about keto and create your own vegetarian dishes!

Eating Out

There's no doubt that doing keto is easiest in your own home, where you have complete control over everything you eat. However, for most people with busy lives, this simply isn't realistic all the time. I would like to stress here that most of your meals *should* be prepared at home by you, but it is perfectly possible to eat keto when dining out or ordering in.

As a mom of four busy kids and one active puppy, I order food to go about once a week. The secret is knowing what to add, what to take out, and how to decipher a takeout menu. For meat-eating keto followers, their main dish will be mostly meat. But for keto vegetarians, the meal should center on vegetables. Ask for your vegetables to be cooked in butter, and if avocado or cheese can be added, even better.

Keep in mind these three things:

1. Your meal needs to have fat—in a few different forms, if possible. Nuts, cheese, oils, and butters as well as avocado and coconut are great options.

2. Skip the sauces unless they are cream based. Barbecue and teriyaki sauces will be loaded with sugars (i.e., carbs).

3. Keep to the keto-approved list of veggies. Many sit-down restaurants will offer eggs on the side or even tofu for some added protein. Skip the fruits and just enjoy those at home (in moderation and bearing in mind which fruits to eat; see page 8).

Find Support

With every big chapter or change in life, a support system can really help. Let's be frank: Switching your brain to a whole new way of thinking about food can be a bit challenging and takes some getting used to. Chances are not everyone in your life with be 100-percent supportive of your new journey, and that's okay. Even if you are not finding the support you need within your own family or circle of friends, you can find a community of supportive people who will understand. Whether it is an online forum, a Facebook group, or an accountability partner, you will find the challenges and successes easier and more satisfying if you have some like-minded people on your side.

A great way to get people on board, whether it's family, friends, or coworkers, is to share with them the reasons you want to try keto. Maybe you want to lose weight, improve mental clarity, or fight an autoimmune disease. Whatever the reason, when other people understand, they are more likely to be supportive. Eating keto might even provide you with opportunities to explain the science behind it and allow others to learn from you, perhaps inspiring them to make changes in their own life.

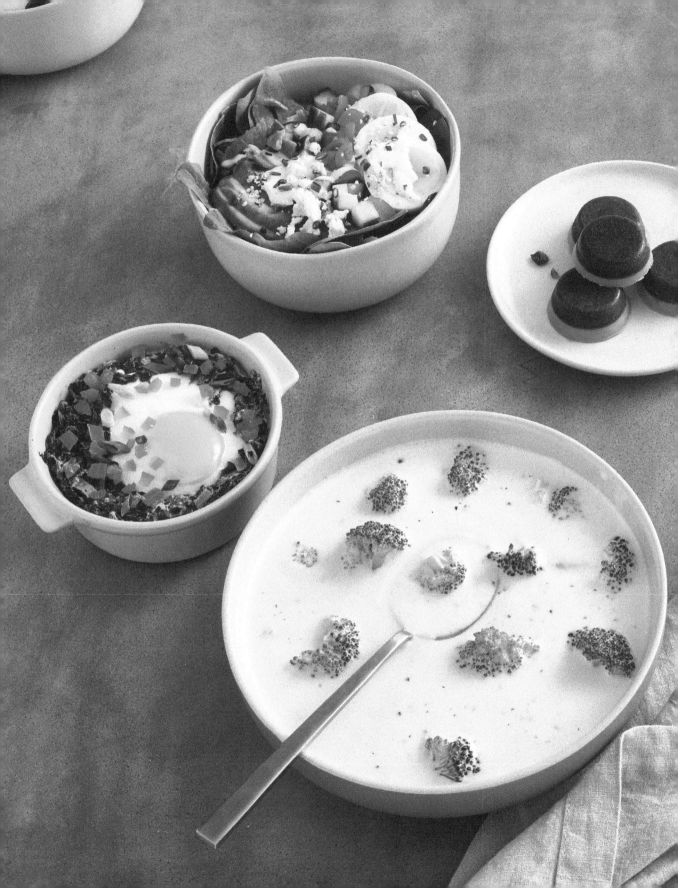

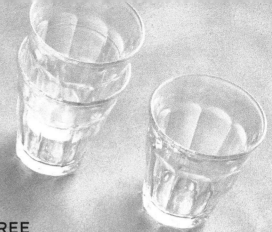

CHAPTER THREE

14-Day Meal Plan
and Beyond

Following a meal plan dramatically increases the odds of successfully sticking to a diet. To get you started, I have created a 14-day meal plan for you to follow. Not only is this plan an effective way to introduce you to vegetarian ketogenic food, but by the end of the 14 days, you should be in ketosis. Whenever I sign up a new client, the first thing I do is create a meal plan for them. This allows them to see exactly what they are supposed to eat, what groceries they are to purchase, and how their meals should be structured. The following 14-day plan gives you just enough variety to make mealtimes interesting but not so many options that you get stuck in the kitchen all day. Each day's dishes combine to give you the correct ratio of macros to get you moving into ketosis.

Shopping List for Week 1

Canned and bottled items

- Olives, black, 1 (6-ounce) can
- Olives, green, 1 (6-ounce) jar
- Marinara sauce, low-sugar, 1 (23-ounce) jar

Dairy and eggs

- Butter, grass-fed, 4 (8-tablespoon) sticks
- Cheddar cheese, sharp (1 pound)
- Cream cheese, 1 (16-ounce) box
- Eggs (1½ dozen)
- Feta cheese, crumbled (14 ounces)
- Greek yogurt, plain full-fat (32 ounces)
- Heavy (whipping) cream (32 ounces)
- Plant-based milk; unsweetened, almond, cashew, or coconut (1 quart)
- Mozzarella cheese, sliced (1 cup)
- Parmesan cheese, 2 (6-ounce) jars
- Pepper Jack cheese, shredded (16 ounces)
- Sour cream (24 ounces)

Frozen foods

- Spinach, 1 (10-ounce) package

Pantry items

- Almond butter
- Avocado oil
- Cashews
- Cinnamon, ground
- Cocoa powder, unsweetened
- Coconut flakes, unsweetened
- Coconut oil
- Coffee, black
- Curry powder
- Dijon mustard
- Garlic powder
- Ginger, ground
- Flaxseeds, ground
- Hemp seeds
- Liquid smoke
- MCT oil (optional)
- Olive oil mayonnaise
- Olive oil
- Onion powder
- Oregano, dried
- Parsley, dried
- Pecans

- Pepitas
- Pepper, black
- Peanut butter, natural, crunchy
- Psyllium husk powder
- Ranch seasoning
- Salt
- Sea salt

- Stevia, liquid
- Sugar-free syrup (I prefer Walden Farms)
- Sunflower seeds
- Vanilla extract
- Veganaise
- Worcestershire sauce

Produce

- Almonds, raw (1 pound)
- Avocados, medium (4)
- Basil (1 bunch)
- Bell pepper (1)
- Butter lettuce (3 heads)
- Cauliflower (1 head)
- Celery (2 stalks)
- Cilantro (1 bunch)
- Cucumbers, medium (2)
- Garlic (1 bulb)
- Kale (1 bunch)

- Lime (1)
- Mushrooms, button (1 pound)
- Onion, white (2)
- Poblano chiles (8)
- Romaine lettuce (4 cups)
- Rosemary, minced (2 tablespoons)
- Salsa (½ cup)
- Spinach (4 cups)
- Thyme (1 bunch)
- Tomatoes, cherry, 1 (14-ounce) container

Other

- BOCA meatless crumbles (2 cups)
- Protein powder (whey or vegan), vanilla (2 tablespoons)

Menus for Week 1

MONDAY

TOTAL MACROS: Fat: 80%; Protein: 12%; Carbs: 8%

BREAKFAST: Fat Coffee

SNACK: Smoked Almonds

LUNCH: Curried Egg Salad

DINNER: Chiles Rellenos

DESSERT: No-Bake Coconut Cookies

TUESDAY

TOTAL MACROS: Fat: 69%; Protein: 20%; Carbs: 11%

BREAKFAST: Kale Refresher Smoothie

SNACK: Baked Olives

LUNCH: Classic Club Salad

DINNER: Cheesy Cauliflower Mac 'n' Cheese

DESSERT: Pecan Pie Pudding

WEDNESDAY

TOTAL MACROS: Fat: 75%; Protein: 14%; Carbs: 11%

BREAKFAST: Superfood Granola

SNACK: Creamy Spinach Dip

LUNCH: Taco Lettuce Cups

DINNER: Margherita Pizza

DESSERT: "Frosty" Chocolate Shake

THURSDAY

TOTAL MACROS: Fat: 80%; Protein: 12%; Carbs: 8%

BREAKFAST: Fat Coffee

SNACK: Smoked Almonds

LUNCH: Curried Egg Salad

DINNER: Chiles Rellenos

DESSERT: No-Bake Coconut Cookies

FRIDAY

TOTAL MACROS: Fat: 69%; Protein: 20%; Carbs: 11%

BREAKFAST: Kale Refresher Smoothie

SNACK: Baked Olives

LUNCH: Classic Club Salad

DINNER: Cheesy Cauliflower Mac 'n' Cheese

DESSERT: Pecan Pie Pudding

SATURDAY

TOTAL MACROS: Fat: 80%; Protein: 12%; Carbs: 8%

BREAKFAST: Fat Coffee

SNACK: Smoked Almonds

LUNCH: Curried Egg Salad

DINNER: Chiles Rellenos

DESSERT: No-Bake Coconut Cookies

SUNDAY

TOTAL MACROS: Fat: 75%; Protein: 14%; Carbs: 11%

BREAKFAST: Superfood Granola

SNACK: Creamy Spinach Dip

LUNCH: Taco Lettuce Cups

DINNER: Margherita Pizza

DESSERT: "Frosty" Chocolate Shake

Shopping List for Week 2

Canned and bottled items

- Coconut milk, full-fat, 5 (14-ounce) cans
- Olives, black, 1 (6-ounce) can
- Tomatoes, diced 1 (14-ounce) can

Dairy and eggs

- Butter, grass-fed, 2 (8-tablespoon) sticks
- Cheddar cheese, shredded (3 cups)
- Cream cheese, 3 (16-ounce) boxes
- Eggs (1 dozen)
- Greek yogurt, 1 (32-ounce) container
- Gruyère cheese (6 slices)
- Heavy (whipping) cream, 1 (16-ounce) container
- Plant-based milk; cashew, almond, or hemp (1 quart)
- Mozzarella cheese, shredded (1 cup)
- Parmesan cheese, 2 (16-ounce) bags
- Provolone cheese (2 slices)

Frozen foods

- Cauliflower rice (or pearls), 1 (10-ounce) box
- Stir-fry vegetables, 1 (20-ounce) bag

Pantry items

- Almonds, dry-roasted
- Almond flour
- Chia seeds
- Dark chocolate chips, low-carb
- Cashews
- Cashew butter, creamy
- Cinnamon, ground
- Cocoa powder, unsweetened
- Coconut aminos, liquid
- Coconut oil
- Cumin, ground
- Curry powder
- Dijon mustard
- Erythritol, granulated
- Erythritol, powdered
- "Everything but the Bagel" seasoning
- Garam masala
- Garlic powder
- MCT powder (optional)
- Olive oil
- Soy sauce

- Peanut butter, creamy, natural
- Pepper, black
- Salt
- Stevia, liquid
- Tamari sauce
- Vanilla extract

Produce

- Avocado, medium (3)
- Basil pesto, 1 (6-ounce) jar
- Bell pepper, green (2)
- Bell pepper, red (2)
- Broccoli, florets (1 cup)
- Cabbage, green, shredded (1 cup)
- Cabbage, purple, shredded (1 cup)
- Cauliflower (2 heads)
- Cilantro (1 bunch)
- Cucumber, medium (3)
- Garlic (1 bulb)
- Ginger (2-inch piece)
- Green beans (14 ounces)
- Kale, chopped (2 cups)
- Lemon (1)
- Lettuce, iceberg (1 head)
- Lime (1)
- Onion, white (1)
- Onion, yellow (1)
- Scallions (1 bunch)
- Strawberries (1 cup)
- Parsley, flat leaf (1 bunch)
- Pickles (1 jar)
- Zucchini, large (2)

Other

- Keto bread (see recipe on page 143)
- Protein powder, vanilla (2 tablespoons)
- Shirataki noodles (3 cups)
- Tofu (10 ounces)

Menus for Week 2

MONDAY

TOTAL MACROS: Fat: 83%; Protein: 8%; Carbs: 9%

BREAKFAST: Fat Hot Chocolate

SNACK: Mediterranean Cucumber Bites

LUNCH: Avocado Pesto Panini

DINNER: Vegan Coconut Curry

DESSERT: Keto Cheesecake

TUESDAY

TOTAL MACROS: Fat: 70%; Protein: 13%; Carbs: 17%

BREAKFAST: Creamy Snickerdoodle Shake

SNACK: Cheesy Crackers

LUNCH: Thai Noodle Salad

DINNER: Kale and Cashew Stir-Fry

DESSERT: Chocolate Peanut Butter Cups

WEDNESDAY

TOTAL MACROS: Fat: 67%; Protein: 21%; Carbs: 12%

BREAKFAST: Broccoli Quiche

SNACK: "Everything but the Bagel" Fat Bombs

LUNCH: Loaded Bell Pepper Sandwich

DINNER: Tofu Green Bean Casserole

DESSERT: Chocolate Sea Salt Almonds

THURSDAY

TOTAL MACROS: Fat: 83%; Protein: 8%; Carbs: 9%

BREAKFAST: Fat Hot Chocolate

SNACK: Mediterranean Cucumber Bites

LUNCH: Avocado Pesto Panini

DINNER: Vegan Coconut Curry

DESSERT: Keto Cheesecake

FRIDAY

TOTAL MACROS: Fat: 70%; Protein: 13%; Carbs: 17%

BREAKFAST: Creamy Snickerdoodle Shake

SNACK: Cheesy Crackers

LUNCH: Thai Noodle Salad

DINNER: Kale and Cashew Stir-Fry

DESSERT: Chocolate Peanut Butter Cups

SATURDAY

TOTAL MACROS: Fat: 83%; Protein: 8%; Carbs: 9%

BREAKFAST: Fat Hot Chocolate

SNACK: Mediterranean Cucumber Bites

LUNCH: Avocado Pesto Panini

DINNER: Vegan Coconut Curry

DESSERT: Keto Cheesecake

SUNDAY

TOTAL MACROS: Fat: 67%; Protein: 21%; Carbs: 12%

BREAKFAST: Broccoli Quiche

SNACK: "Everything but the Bagel" Fat Bombs

LUNCH: Loaded Bell Pepper Sandwich

DINNER: Tofu Green Bean Casserole

DESSERT: Chocolate Sea Salt Almonds

The Keto-Adapted Life

The term "keto-adapted" simply means your body has found a good balance with ketosis and is producing ketones naturally. Once you become keto-adapted, your body will continue to burn fat night and day. Going forward, you have a few options. If your energy is good, your satiation level feels about right, and you are seeing results, stay on track. Remain consistent with your calorie count and macro percentages. However, if you find that you're getting hungry, try raising your calorie intake by 100 calories per day for a week. If you are still hungry after that week, add another 100 calories per day, but make sure to keep the macro percentages the same. If you aren't seeing results or have reached a plateau, you can add one 24-hour fasting day per week as well as really concentrate on eating all your fats. Remember that if you aren't paying attention to the details, such as counting your macros, you most likely won't be seeing the results you want to see.

Adjust as Needed

When my clients begin to see signs of success, I always remind them that I am only half of the equation. That also applies to this book. I have done the easy part by sharing the fundamentals of keto, but the rest is up to you. Hopefully you will stick to the plan and experience some great results. This method of eating is easy to tailor for the long term, and you may even continue to see improvements over time. Maybe your initial goal was weight loss and reduced inflammation, but after some time in keto, you realize that you also really enjoy the mental clarity and reduced sugar cravings that come with stable blood sugar. Many people also notice that eating keto long term calms their digestive system as well.

The key to following any plan for an extended period of time is finding a happy balance, and no diet should control your life, so embrace a certain amount of flexibility. For example, you may have a trip coming up and you want to enjoy unfamiliar foods. That's okay: Make a plan to be off keto throughout your trip, and then when you have returned home and feel ready, do the work to get back into ketosis. Life is meant to be lived, and if you can come to terms with that, you will be in good shape.

Cheat Days

The term "cheat day" has become very popular. It refers to taking a small break from your current diet by eating something not included in your plan. Most people on a typical calorie-restrictive diet can enjoy a cheat day and then jump right back on track the next day.

With keto, however, cheat days can be a bit tricky. With keto, either you are in ketosis or you are not. And just one carb-filled meal can knock you right out of ketosis. Getting back into ketosis is not easy. It takes work. So, cheat days might not be worth it.

Here is something important to consider when you start dreaming of cheating: It will most likely make you sick, with a stomachache at best and intestinal distress at worst. Your body has become unaccustomed to processing carbs as it used to, and while you will most likely enjoy the first few bites, shortly afterward you will most likely regret it.

Can you ever have a cheat meal on keto? (Notice I did not say cheat *day*, just one meal.) Yes, a cheat meal is possible, but be patient. You can try introducing one cheat meal per week, but only after you have been on the ketogenic diet for at least four weeks. Start with a fairly small portion and see how your body handles it. The next week, increase your cheat meal plate ever so slightly to avoid getting sick.

FALLING OFF THE KETO WAGON

Diving off the keto deep end into a banana split followed by some French fries and a giant cinnamon roll can happen. And it's okay. You don't have to be 100-percent perfect all the time; slippage can happen. What you are doing and have done is hard, so give yourself the credit you deserve for deciding to take control of your life and health, and get back on the wagon.

On a positive note, once you have been keto-adapted, it is easier to get back into ketosis. The first thing to do after a slip is to start your next keto cycle with a 24-hour fast. Then be sure to add exogenous ketones to your water. These are a supplemental form of the ketones naturally produced by the body and will help you bounce back into keto as fast as possible and stay there. After that, add as many keto-approved fats as possible and resume the daily tracking of your macro percentages. Test every night for ketones, and once you hit those numbers, you are on your way to burning fat again.

Staying Healthy

When considering any new eating plan, it is very important to schedule an appointment with your primary doctor and go over any questions or concerns you have, and the same is true of the keto diet. Ask for a blood panel to be done so you have a baseline. This bloodwork can be repeated 30, 60, or 90 days after you have become keto-adapted. Your doctor will most likely give you advice on any supplements that should be added to your diet as well as how to maintain your cardiac health and keep your cholesterol levels in check. Also, if you are prediabetic or diabetic, you will need to pay careful attention to your glucose numbers.

Exercise is always a good option on keto. Listen to your body as much as possible; it's very clever at telling you what it needs. In the first week or two of getting your body into ketosis, you will most likely be lacking in energy. Don't force it. Use this time to do some yoga or light stretching or go for walks. Your body will be under some stress, so until you reach ketosis, don't feel that you have to stress your body more by engaging in intense workouts. However, once you are keto-adapted, stay as active as possible, even adding some of your favorite workouts. Plenty of people have run marathons, won bodybuilding competitions, and even completed Ironman races while in ketosis.

Get Creative in the Kitchen

Once you've mastered the recipes in this book, you will have all the skills you need to continue your vegetarian ketogenic way of life. The recipes are my idea of what possibilities there are for a vegetarian on keto, but it's probable that you will have your own preferences and ideas for meals and flavor combinations to try. While trying out my recipes, you can start to brainstorm about which keto-friendly ingredients you want to eat more of. Chances are you will discover at least a few new favorite dishes from this book, and you can also adapt some of your current recipes to be more keto compliant. My motto has always been Eat Good, Feel Good, and Look Good, and I have no doubt you will experience all three of these benefits from a vegetarian keto lifestyle. There is a lot to be said for being able to enjoy the food you love and knowing it is good for you!

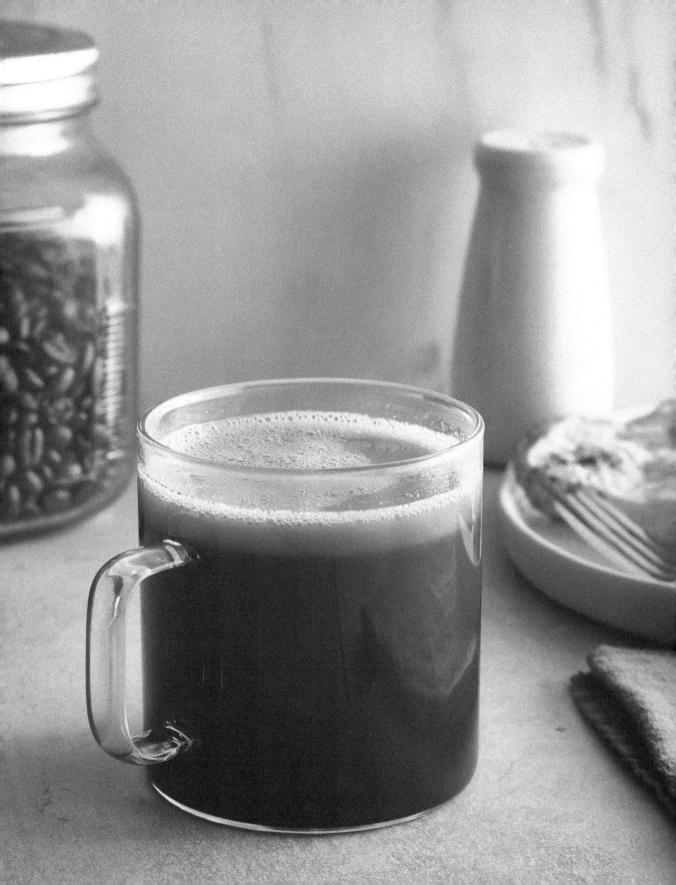

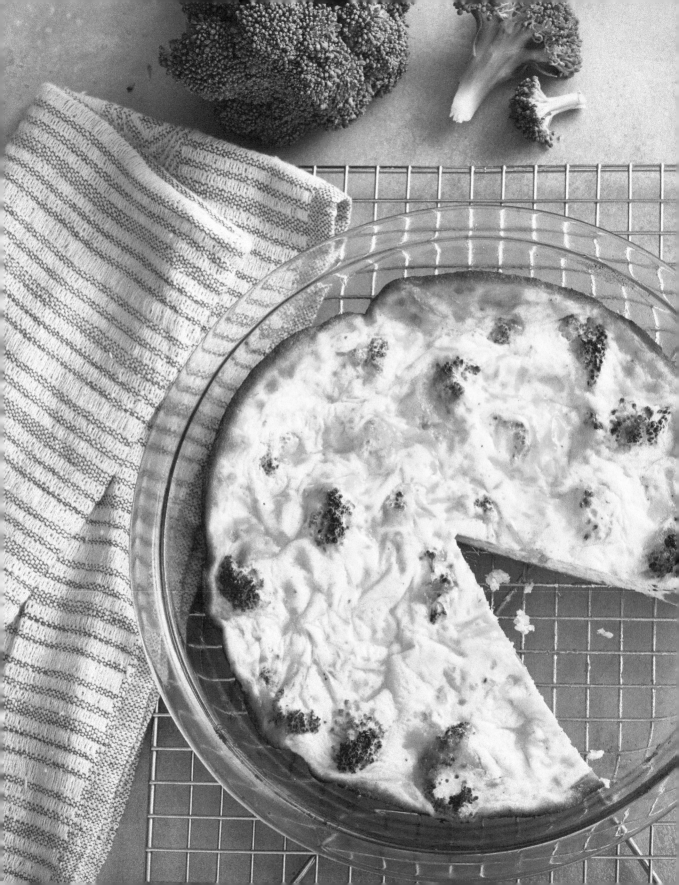

CHAPTER FOUR

Breakfast and Smoothies

Kale Refresher Smoothie 32

Spirulina Smoothie 33

Fat Drinks Three Ways 34

Matcha Coffee 36

Creamy Snickerdoodle Shake 37

Superfood Granola 38

Creamed Spinach with Eggs 39

Mexican Egg Casserole 40

Italian Vegetable Egg Bake 42

Eggs Benedict with Five-Minute Hollandaise 43

▶ Broccoli Quiche 44

Almond Butter Pancakes 45

Zucchini Chocolate Muffins 46

Coconut Flaxseed Waffles 47

Chocolate Coconut "Oatmeal" 48

Cream Cheese Pumpkin Muffins 49

KALE REFRESHER SMOOTHIE

DAIRY-FREE, EGG-FREE, GLUTEN-FREE
Serves 1 / Prep time: 5 minutes

This green smoothie will kick-start your day on the right foot. It is loaded with healthy fats perfect for keto, such as hemp seeds, avocado, and coconut oil, and keeps the micronutrients high with iron-rich kale. Adding the perfect amount of protein powder will help with muscle recovery if you want to use this recipe as a post-workout meal.

1 cup unsweetened almond, cashew, or coconut milk

½ medium cucumber, peeled and halved lengthwise

1 tablespoon vanilla protein powder (whey or vegan)

½ lime, peeled and deseeded

1 tablespoon hemp seeds

1 avocado, sliced

1 cup frozen kale, stems removed

1 tablespoon coconut oil, melted

5 to 6 stevia drops

1 cup ice cubes

1. In a high-powered blender, combine the milk, cucumber, protein powder, lime, hemp seeds, avocado, kale, and coconut oil. Blend for 30 seconds.

2. Add the stevia and ice cubes, and then blend on high for 1 minute.

3. Pour into a glass and serve.

Prep tip: This is a great meal to prep ahead of time. Put all the ingredients except the milk and ice in a resealable freezer bag and freeze for up to 4 weeks. Before blending, remove the ingredients from the bag and add the milk and ice.

Per Serving (1 smoothie) **Calories:** 634; Fat: 46g; Protein: 21g; Total carbs: 32g; Net carbs: 14g; Fiber: 18g; Sugar: 4g; Sodium: 252mg **Macros:** Fat: 65%; Protein: 15%; Carbs: 20%

SPIRULINA SMOOTHIE

DAIRY-FREE, EGG-FREE, GLUTEN-FREE
Serves 1 / Prep time: 5 minutes

Flaxseed is a great addition to this smoothie due to its high omega-3 and fiber content. It can also help improve cholesterol levels as well as reduce the risk of heart disease. When flaxseed is paired with another superfood such as spirulina, the health benefits are endless.

1 cup full-fat coconut milk

1 tablespoon coconut cream

1 teaspoon finely diced fresh ginger

½ teaspoon spirulina powder

¼ teaspoon ground cardamom

¼ teaspoon ground cinnamon

1 tablespoon vanilla protein powder
 (vegan or whey)

1 cup ice cubes

1 teaspoon flaxseed

1. In a high-powered blender, combine the coconut milk, coconut cream, ginger, spirulina, cardamom, and cinnamon. Blend for 30 seconds.

2. Add the protein powder and ice cubes, and blend on high for 1 minute.

3. Pour the smoothie into a glass, sprinkle the flaxseed on top, and enjoy.

Ingredient tip: Coconut cream may be referred to as coconut concentrate or cream of coconut. It should be easy to find at local health food stores, but if you cannot find it, you can use the top layer of cream from a can of coconut milk instead.

Per Serving (1 smoothie) **Calories:** 708; Fat: 60g; Protein: 15g; Total carbs: 27g; Net carbs: 20g; Fiber: 7g; Sugar: 18g; Sodium: 81mg **Macros:** Fat: 77%; Protein: 8%; Carbs: 15%

FAT DRINKS THREE WAYS

These drinks may well likely become your morning keto staples. I've included three different recipes to keep your taste buds excited and get you on your way to nutritional ketosis. Drinking one of these at least five days a week is a quick way to get a good amount of fat into your diet without spending the morning cooking.

FAT COFFEE

EGG-FREE, GLUTEN-FREE, NUT-FREE
Serves 1 / Prep time: 5 minutes / Cook time: 5 minutes

8 to 12 ounces black coffee

1 tablespoon grass-fed butter

1 to 2 tablespoons MCT oil (or powder) or
   coconut oil

Pinch sea salt

1. Pour the coffee into a small saucepan over medium heat.

2. Stir in the butter, MCT oil, and salt.

3. Warm the mixture slowly, continuing to stir for 3 to 4 minutes, and then serve warm.

Prep tip: If you make your coffee first thing in the morning, you can skip to stirring in the butter and oil right in your mug.

Per Serving (1 drink) **Calories:** 221; Fat: 25g; Protein: 0g; Total carbs: 0g; Net carbs: 0g; Fiber: 0g; Sugar: 0g; Sodium: 286mg **Macros:** Fat: 99%; Protein: 1%; Carbs: 0%

FAT HOT CHOCOLATE

EGG-FREE, GLUTEN-FREE
Serves 1 / Prep time: 5 minutes / Cook time: 5 minutes

2 tablespoons cocoa powder

8 ounces plant-based milk (cashew, almond,
   or hemp)

2 tablespoons heavy (whipping) cream

1 tablespoon coconut oil or MCT powder

1 tablespoon grass-fed butter

5 to 6 drops liquid stevia (optional)

1. In a small saucepan over medium heat, combine the cocoa powder, milk, cream, coconut oil, and butter.

2. Stir continuously for 3 to 4 minutes until the mixture is warm.

3. Remove the pan from the heat, and stir in the stevia (if using). Serve warm.

Leftovers tip: Double this batch and store the remainder in a thermos in the refrigerator. This can make for a quick grab-and-go meal on a busy morning. When reheating, pour the mixture into a glass measuring cup and heat in the microwave for 90 seconds. Give it a good stir and enjoy!

Per Serving (1 drink) **Calories:** 371; Fat: 39g; Protein: 2g; Total carbs: 3g; Net carbs: 2g; Fiber: 1g; Sugar: 0g; Sodium: 257mg **Macros:** Fat: 95%; Protein: 2%; Carbs: 3%

FAT CHAI

EGG-FREE, GLUTEN-FREE
Serves 1 / Prep time: 5 minutes / Cook time: 5 minutes

2 sugar-free chai tea bags

8 to 12 ounces hot water

1 tablespoon coconut oil

1 tablespoon grass-fed butter

2 tablespoons heavy (whipping) cream

5 to 6 drops of stevia (optional)

1. Steep both tea bags in the hot water for 5 minutes.

2. Remove the tea bags and stir in the coconut oil, butter, and cream. Stir until well blended.

3. Stir in the stevia (if using) and serve warm.

Ingredient tip: If you have trouble finding sugar-free chai tea bags at your local grocery store, try making your own spice mix. Combine 2 teaspoons ground cinnamon, 1 teaspoon ground ginger, ½ teaspoon ground cardamom, and ¼ teaspoon ground cloves.

Per Serving (1 drink) **Calories:** 323; Fat: 35g; Protein: 1g; Total carbs: 1g; Net carbs: 1g; Fiber: 0g; Sugar: 0g; Sodium: 93mg **Macros:** Fat: 98%; Protein: 1%; Carbs: 1%

MATCHA COFFEE

DAIRY-FREE, EGG-FREE, GLUTEN-FREE
Serves 2 / Prep time: 5 minutes

Matcha tea is regarded by many as the "superfood of all superfoods." It is less processed than regular green tea, meaning it contains more vitamins, minerals, protein, and antioxidants. One protein it includes is L-theanine, which helps create a slow-releasing, caffeine-like buzz. Many premade matcha drinks contain high amounts of sugar, but with this keto-friendly recipe, you'll be well on your way to ketosis.

1 (13.5-ounce) can full-fat coconut milk

1 cup brewed black coffee, chilled

1 tablespoon almond butter

2 teaspoons matcha powder, plus more for sprinkling

1 cup ice cubes

5 to 6 drops liquid stevia or monk fruit

1. In a high-powered blender, combine the coconut milk, coffee, almond butter, matcha powder, ice, and stevia, and blend on high speed for 60 seconds.

2. Divide the drink between two glasses and sprinkle each with a bit more matcha powder.

Ingredient tip: Not all matcha powders are created equal, which is reflected in the variation in cost (anywhere from $2 to $2,000 an ounce). The good news is that the more affordable powders can be found at your local grocery stores and are excellent for this recipe.

Per Serving (1 drink) **Calories:** 508; Fat: 48g; Protein: 7g; Total carbs: 12g; Net carbs: 7g; Fiber: 5g; Sugar: 7g; Sodium: 65mg **Macros:** Fat: 85%; Protein: 6%; Carbs: 9%

CREAMY SNICKERDOODLE SHAKE

DAIRY-FREE, EGG-FREE, GLUTEN-FREE
Serves 2 / Prep time: 5 minutes

Snickerdoodle has been a classic comfort flavor for generations. Any diet will be much easier to stick with if you can keep enjoying wonderful flavors in your meals. The coconut-milk base of the smoothie gives a lovely creamy texture to this cinnamon concoction.

1 cup full-fat coconut milk

1 cup water

1 teaspoon ground cinnamon

2 tablespoons chia seeds

2 tablespoons coconut oil

1 scoop vanilla protein powder

1. In a high-powered blender, combine the coconut milk, water, cinnamon, chia seeds, coconut oil, and protein powder and blend on high for 60 seconds.

2. Divide the shake between two glasses and enjoy.

Change it up: For a thicker shake, use only ½ cup of water. For another variation, add 2 tablespoons of cacao powder and 1 tablespoon of almond butter.

Per Serving (1 drink) **Calories:** 535; Fat: 47g; Protein: 13g; Total carbs: 15g; Net carbs: 6g; Fiber: 9g; Sugar: 4g; Sodium: 45mg **Macros:** Fat: 79%; Protein: 10%; Carbs: 11%

SUPERFOOD GRANOLA

DAIRY-FREE, EGG-FREE, GLUTEN-FREE
Serves 2 / Prep time: 5 minutes / Cook time: 20 minutes

With plenty of heart-healthy seeds and coconut, this granola is a perfect example of how you can transform foods that would normally be off-limits into keto-friendly favorites. Try topping a bowl of it with Greek yogurt for a morning parfait. It's an easy recipe to double so you'll have a healthy, tasty breakfast ready for the next morning.

½ cup unsweetened coconut flakes

2 tablespoons ground flaxseed

2 tablespoons pepitas

2 tablespoons sunflower seeds

3 tablespoons chopped pecans

2 tablespoons coconut oil, melted

1 teaspoon ground cinnamon

½ teaspoon ground ginger

1 teaspoon salt

1. Preheat the oven to 350°F.

2. In a medium bowl, combine the coconut flakes, flaxseed, pepitas, sunflower seeds, and pecans, and mix well.

3. Pour the coconut oil over the mixture and stir to coat well. Sprinkle with the cinnamon, ginger, and salt and stir for about 1 minute until well combined.

4. Spread the granola on a rimmed baking sheet and bake for 20 minutes, tossing the granola every 3 to 4 minutes.

5. Remove the baking sheet from the oven once the mixture is light golden brown, and set aside to cool thoroughly.

Leftovers tip: The granola can be stored in a resealable quart-size bag or airtight container for up to 1 week.

Per Serving **Calories:** 377; Fat: 35g; Protein: 6g; Total carbs: 10g; Net carbs: 3g; Fiber: 7g; Sugar: 1g; Sodium: 1169mg **Macros:** Fat: 84%; Protein: 6%; Carbs: 10%

CREAMED SPINACH WITH EGGS

GLUTEN-FREE
Serves 4 / Prep time: 10 minutes / Cook time: 15 minutes

This traditional holiday dish can be enjoyed all year, for any meal of the day. It showcases the wonderful taste and aroma of nutmeg, which touts some pretty amazing health benefits such as helping lower cholesterol, improving memory, and even keeping gums healthy. The fried eggs add some fat to burn ketones.

2 tablespoons grass-fed butter

8 eggs

Nonstick cooking spray

½ cup finely diced white onion

2 garlic cloves, minced

1½ tablespoons almond flour

1½ cups unsweetened almond milk

2 tablespoons grated Parmesan cheese

4 ounces Greek yogurt cream cheese

¾ teaspoon salt

½ teaspoon freshly ground black pepper

¼ teaspoon ground nutmeg

16 ounces frozen spinach, thawed, drained, and squeezed dry

1. Heat a large griddle over medium-high heat. Melt the butter, and then crack the eggs into the pan. Reduce the heat to low and cook slowly until the egg whites begin to thicken. Slide a spatula under each egg and carefully flip it over. Cook for another 3 to 4 minutes. Remove from the heat and set aside.

2. Spray a large skillet with cooking spray. Over medium heat, soften the onion and garlic in the skillet for about 4 minutes.

3. Whisk in the almond flour and cook for an additional minute.

4. Reduce the heat to low and whisk in the milk, Parmesan cheese, Greek yogurt cream cheese, salt, pepper, and nutmeg. Mix until completely smooth.

5. Add the spinach and combine well with the sauce. Cook for 1 more minute, or until the spinach is heated through.

6. Place the fried eggs on top of the creamed spinach and divide into 4 equal servings.

Change it up: For a baked, single-serving variation, divide the spinach mixture into 8 small ramekins, crack an egg on top of each one, and bake at 375°F for 20 minutes.

Per Serving **Calories:** 345; Fat: 25g; Protein: 20g; Total carbs: 11g; Net carbs: 7g; Fiber: 4g; Sugar: 2g; Sodium: 911mg **Macros:** Fat: 65%; Protein: 23%; Carbs: 12%

MEXICAN EGG CASSEROLE

GLUTEN-FREE

Serves 8 / Prep time: 15 minutes / Cook time: 45 minutes

Some people used to eating a meat-free diet struggle with the vegetarian keto diet's reliance on eggs. This dish is a great way to ease into the diet, thanks to its volume of veggies. It's a quick and easy dish to throw together on busy mornings (or nights!). If you're cooking for a crowd of meat eaters, you can easily make an extra batch with some chopped ham or sausage.

Nonstick cooking spray

2 tablespoons olive oil

1 cup chopped green bell pepper

½ cup minced onion

2 garlic cloves, minced

3 cups raw spinach

Salt

Freshly ground black pepper

½ cup unsweetened almond milk

12 eggs

1½ cups grated cheddar cheese, divided

1 avocado, sliced

1 cup salsa

1. Preheat the oven to 375°F. Spray a nonstick 9-by-13-inch casserole dish with cooking spray and set aside.

2. In a skillet over medium-high heat, warm the olive oil. Add the bell pepper, onion, and garlic, and sauté for about 3 minutes. Then add the spinach and allow to wilt. Season with a pinch of salt and pepper. Remove the skillet from the heat and set aside.

3. In a medium bowl, whisk together the milk, eggs, and 1 cup of cheddar cheese.

4. Spread the veggies out in the casserole dish and pour the egg mixture on top.

5. Top with the remaining ½ cup of cheddar cheese.

6. Set the dish in the oven and bake for 40 minutes, or until the edges of the casserole are brown and the eggs are set.

7. Divide the casserole between eight plates.

8. Top with the avocado slices and salsa, and serve warm or cold.

Leftovers tip: This dish is a useful meal to keep on hand in the freezer. Assemble the casserole in an 9-by-13-inch aluminum pan and freeze after step five. To reheat, thaw overnight in the refrigerator and bake as directed.

Per Serving **Calories:** 271; Fat: 21g; Protein: 15g; Total carbs: 7g; Net carbs: 4g; Fiber: 3g; Sugar: 3g; Sodium: 472mg **Macros:** Fat: 70%; Protein: 22%; Carbs: 8%

ITALIAN VEGETABLE EGG BAKE

GLUTEN-FREE, NUT-FREE

Serves 4 / Prep time: 10 minutes / Cook time: 30 minutes

Olives are an excellent ingredient for anyone on a keto diet. They contain more nutrients than olive oil, are high in fat, and provide some protein as well. They are also high in micronutrients such as copper and iron, which are great for sustaining energy. Olives come in many different sizes and colors, so choose the ones you like the best.

Nonstick cooking spray

1 (10-ounce) package frozen spinach, thawed, drained, and squeezed dry

1/3 cup diced red bell pepper

1 garlic clove, minced

1 tablespoon minced fresh parsley

3/4 cup diced and drained canned artichokes

1 cup black olives, sliced

1/2 cup diced scallions

1/4 teaspoon cayenne pepper

12 eggs

1/4 cup heavy (whipping) cream

1 1/4 teaspoons salt

1/2 teaspoon freshly ground black pepper

1. Preheat the oven to 375°F. Spray a 9-by-13-inch baking dish with cooking spray and set aside.

2. In a small bowl, combine the spinach, bell pepper, garlic, parsley, artichokes, olives, and scallions. Stir well. Add the cayenne pepper and mix until the vegetables are well coated.

3. Spread the vegetables in the bottom of the prepared baking dish.

4. In a separate bowl, whisk together the eggs, cream, salt, and black pepper. Pour the egg mixture over the vegetables.

5. Bake for 30 minutes, or until the eggs are set.

6. Remove the dish from the oven and let stand for about 7 minutes before serving.

Change it up: When substituting ingredients, it is important to keep the items low-carb and high-fat so that you can stay in ketosis. You can get creative and add other vegetables such as zucchini, mushrooms, or broccoli, but avoid starchier vegetables, such as sweet potatoes, peas, or corn, as they would likely kick you out of ketosis.

Per Serving **Calories:** 337; Fat: 23g; Protein: 20g; Total carbs: 10g; Net carbs: 6g; Fiber: 4g; Sugar: 3g; Sodium: 511mg **Macros:** Fat: 61%; Protein: 24%; Carbs: 15%

EGGS BENEDICT WITH FIVE-MINUTE HOLLANDAISE

GLUTEN-FREE, NUT-FREE
Serves 2 / Prep time: 10 minutes / Cook time: 20 minutes

Hollandaise is traditionally known as one of the "mother" sauces in French cuisine, but here in the States we know it as an extravagant topping for eggs Benedict. Typically, this dish is served with English muffins and poached eggs, but for the keto version, you'll make it in a vegan-bacon basket (I like Lightlife) and top it with a super-simple hollandaise.

Nonstick cooking spray

4 slices vegan bacon

4 eggs, plus 3 egg yolks

½ cup grass-fed butter (1 stick)

Juice of ½ lemon

⅛ teaspoon cayenne pepper

Chopped fresh parsley, for serving

1 avocado, pitted and sliced, for serving

1. Preheat the oven to 350°F. Spray 4 cups of a muffin tin generously with cooking spray.

2. Line each muffin cup with a strip of bacon, covering the sides as much as possible.

3. Break 1 egg into each bacon nest.

4. Bake the egg cups for 15 to 20 minutes, until the eggs are set in the center.

5. While the eggs are cooking, melt the butter in a cup in the microwave for 30 to 40 seconds.

6. In a blender, combine the egg yolks, lemon juice, and cayenne. With the blender on the lowest speed, slowly drizzle the melted butter into the blender until it is thoroughly combined.

7. Remove the egg cups from the oven and carefully remove each egg basket from the muffin tin.

8. Drizzle the hollandaise sauce over the eggs. Sprinkle each cup with parsley and top with a few avocado slices.

Prep tip: You can use aluminum-foil muffin liners, coated with cooking spray, to ensure that the egg and bacon baskets stay together.

Per Serving (2 egg cups) **Calories:** 822; Fat: 78g; Protein: 19g; Total carbs: 11g; Net carbs: 4g; Fiber: 7g; Sugar: 2g; Sodium: 645mg **Macros:** Fat: 85%; Protein: 9%; Carbs: 6%

BROCCOLI QUICHE

GLUTEN-FREE, NUT-FREE
Serves 2 / Prep time: 10 minutes / Cook time: 30 minutes

Quiche dishes traditionally have a thick crust and combine eggs with various fillings. In this crustless keto version, broccoli takes center stage, with yogurt and cheese providing complementary tanginess. It's a filling option that's easy to make ahead of time in preparation for busy mornings.

Nonstick cooking spray

1 egg, plus 5 egg whites

½ cup plain nonfat Greek yogurt

1 teaspoon salt

¼ teaspoon freshly ground black pepper

1 tablespoon minced garlic

1 cup broccoli florets

1 cup shredded cheddar cheese

1. Preheat the oven to 400°F. Spray a 9-inch pie dish with cooking spray.

2. In a medium bowl, mix together the egg, egg whites, Greek yogurt, salt, pepper, and garlic.

3. Fold in the broccoli and cheddar cheese.

4. Pour the mixture into the prepared pie dish and bake for 30 minutes, or until the eggs are set.

5. Remove the quiche from the oven and allow it to cool for a few minutes before serving.

Prep Tip: This quiche will be thin, so don't wait for it to puff up. Think of it more as a broccoli crêpe that you could even roll up to eat.

Per Serving **Calories:** 352; Fat: 21g; Protein: 33g; Total carbs: 8g; Net carbs: 7g; Fiber: 1g; Sugar: 3g; Sodium: 1663mg **Macros:** Fat: 54%; Protein: 38%; Carbs: 8%

ALMOND BUTTER PANCAKES

DAIRY-FREE, EGG-FREE, GLUTEN-FREE
Serves 1 / **Prep time: 5 minutes** / **Cook time: 10 minutes**

The carb content of pancakes usually makes them a no-no on keto, but here is a wonderful version that you can enjoy without guilt. The high fat content comes from almond butter and grass-fed butter, and regular flour is replaced with a low-carb version.

Nonstick cooking spray

2 tablespoons almond butter

¼ cup unsweetened cashew milk

5 or 6 drops liquid stevia

1 tablespoon ground flaxseed

1 tablespoon coconut flour

½ teaspoon baking powder

½ teaspoon ground cinnamon

2 tablespoons grass-fed butter

1. Spray a skillet with nonstick cooking spray.

2. In a small bowl, combine the almond butter, cashew milk, and stevia.

3. In a separate small bowl, combine the flaxseed, coconut flour, baking powder, and cinnamon. Mix well.

4. Pour the almond-butter-and-milk mixture into the flour mixture and stir until well blended.

5. Allow the batter to sit for 3 to 4 minutes to thicken.

6. Heat the skillet over medium-high heat. When hot, pour the batter into 3- to 4-inch circles and cook for about 4 minutes.

7. Flip the pancakes and cook for an additional 2 minutes.

8. Top with the grass-fed butter and enjoy.

Leftovers tip: Double the batch and freeze half. This is a great way to maximize your time in the kitchen. The pancakes can be stored flat in a resealable quart-size freezer bag in the freezer for up to four weeks.

Per Serving (3 pancakes) **Calories:** 573; Fat: 55g; Protein: 9g; Total carbs: 11g; Net carbs: 4g; Fiber: 7g; Sugar: 1g; Sodium: 288mg **Macros:** Fat: 86%; Protein: 6%; Carbs: 8%

ZUCCHINI CHOCOLATE MUFFINS

DAIRY-FREE, GLUTEN-FREE, NUT-FREE
Makes 12 muffins / Prep time: 5 minutes / Cook time: 15 minutes

Zucchini is one of the shining stars of keto. It's low carb and has fiber in it, which makes it a perfect filler for these muffins. The coconut oil adds a subtle flavor while making the muffins super moist. Low-carb chocolate chips (I recommend Lily's) add a final decadent touch.

3 eggs, beaten

2 cups shredded zucchini

½ cup cacao powder

½ cup coconut oil, slightly melted

1 teaspoon vanilla extract

⅓ cup granulated erythritol

2 tablespoons low-carb dark
  chocolate chips

1. Preheat the oven to 250°F.

2. Grease the cups of a muffin tin (or use liners).

3. In a medium bowl, mix together the eggs, zucchini, cacao powder, coconut oil, vanilla, and erythritol.

4. Pour the batter evenly into the 12 muffin cups.

5. Sprinkle the chocolate chips on the tops of the muffins.

6. Bake for about 15 minutes, or until a knife inserted into the middle of a muffin comes out clean.

7. Transfer the muffins to a cooling rack.

Ingredient tip: If you have a hard time finding low-carb chocolate chips, cacao nibs make a great substitute.

Per Serving (makes 4 servings) **Calories:** 379; Fat: 35g; Protein: 7g; Total carbs: 9g; Net carbs: 5g; Fiber: 4g; Sugar: 1g; Sodium: 54mg; Erythritol carbs: 6g **Macros:** Fat: 83%; Protein: 7%; Carbs: 10%

COCONUT FLAXSEED WAFFLES

GLUTEN-FREE, NUT-FREE

Serves 4 / Prep time: 15 minutes / Cook time: 5 minutes

Re-creating familiar and favorite foods can make the transition from a carb-based diet to a ketogenic diet much easier. These heart-healthy waffles are packed with ingredients that'll fill you up and keep your ketones high.

Nonstick cooking spray

5 eggs

½ cup water

⅓ cup coconut oil, melted

2 cups ground flaxseed

1 tablespoon baking powder

1 teaspoon salt

2 tablespoons unsweetened coconut flakes

5 to 6 drops liquid stevia

4 tablespoons grass-fed butter

1. Spray a waffle iron with cooking spray and heat it to a medium-high temperature. Allow ample time for it to get up to temperature.

2. Combine the eggs, water, and coconut oil in a blender. Blend on high speed for 30 to 40 seconds.

3. In a medium bowl, mix together the flaxseed, baking powder, and salt until combined.

4. Pour the blender mixture into the flaxseed blend and stir. Allow to sit for 4 to 5 minutes to thicken.

5. Add the coconut flakes and stevia, and then mix well to combine.

6. Pour ¼ cup of batter for each waffle onto the waffle iron and allow to cook thoroughly. Repeat until all the batter has been used.

7. Top each waffle with 1 tablespoon of grass-fed butter.

Leftover tip: Because this recipe makes three extra waffles, you can store them in a resealable plastic bag until ready to use. They can be frozen for up to 4 weeks.

Per Serving (1 waffle) **Calories:** 498; Fat: 46g; Protein: 12g; Total carbs: 9g; Net carbs: 2g; Fiber: 7g; Sugar: 0g; Sodium: 162mg **Macros:** Fat: 83%; Protein: 10%; Carbs: 7%

CHOCOLATE COCONUT "OATMEAL"

DAIRY-FREE, EGG-FREE, GLUTEN-FREE
Serves 2 / Prep time: 5 minutes / Cook time: 5 minutes

There's something especially comforting about a piping-hot bowl of oatmeal on a crisp fall morning. This "oatmeal" pairs perfectly with a Fat Coffee or Chai (page 34) to get your day started on a satisfying note.

½ cup unsweetened coconut flakes

¼ cup hemp hearts

1 tablespoon coconut flour

½ cup water

⅓ cup canned full-fat coconut milk

1 teaspoon vanilla extract

2 teaspoons cacao powder

1 tablespoon almond butter

1 teaspoon low-carb dark chocolate chips

1. In a medium saucepan over medium-high heat, combine the coconut flakes, hemp hearts, coconut flour, water, and coconut milk.

2. Bring the mixture to a boil and allow to cook for 2 minutes while stirring.

3. Remove the pan from the heat and stir in the vanilla, cacao powder, and almond butter.

4. Divide the "oatmeal" between two dishes and sprinkle with the chocolate chips.

Change it up: As you get deeper into keto, you will find that you crave sweets less and less. Try this "oatmeal" unsweetened at first and see how you like it. If you feel that you need it a tad sweeter, add a few drops of liquid stevia.

Per Serving **Calories:** 473; Fat: 37g; Protein: 16g; Total carbs: 19g; Net carbs: 7g; Fiber: 12g; Sugar: 3g; Sodium: 12mg **Macros:** Fat: 70%; Protein: 14%; Carbs: 16%

CREAM CHEESE PUMPKIN MUFFINS

GLUTEN-FREE
Makes 12 muffins / Prep time: 15 minutes / Cook time: 20 minutes

Making keto baked goods is easier than it seems. Oftentimes, the white flour can be replaced with better, lower-carb alternatives, and the sugars can be substituted with low-impact sweeteners such as erythritol, monk fruit, or stevia.

Nonstick cooking spray

½ cup grass-fed butter, at room
  temperature

⅔ cup erythritol, granulated

4 large eggs

¾ cup pumpkin purée

1 teaspoon vanilla extract

1½ cups almond flour

½ cup coconut flour

4 teaspoons baking powder

2 teaspoons pumpkin pie spice

½ teaspoon salt

8 ounces Greek yogurt cream cheese

Stevia

Ground cinnamon

1. Preheat the oven to 350°F. Line the cups of a muffin tin with liners or grease well with cooking spray.

2. Using a stand mixer (or in a large bowl with a hand mixer), mix together the butter and erythritol until creamy.

3. Add the eggs one at a time, mixing thoroughly after the addition of each egg.

4. Stir in the pumpkin and vanilla and mix well.

5. In a small bowl, mix together the almond flour, coconut flour, baking powder, pumpkin pie spice, and salt.

6. Pour the flour mixture into the butter mixture and mix well to combine. Divide the batter evenly between the muffin cups.

7. In a separate small bowl, stir the cream cheese until softened. Add stevia to taste.

8. Top each muffin with about 1 tablespoon of cream cheese. Sprinkle with cinnamon.

9. Bake for about 20 minutes, or until the muffin tops are slightly brown.

Prep tip: This would be a perfect recipe to make on a Sunday to have breakfast prepared for the rest of the week. It's a great grab-and-go option.

Per Serving (2 muffins) **Calories:** 447; Fat: 35g; Protein: 14g; Total carbs: 19g; Net carbs: 12g; Fiber: 7g; Sugar: 1g; Sodium: 367mg; Erythritol carbs: 12g **Macros:** Fat: 70%; Protein: 13%; Carbs: 17%

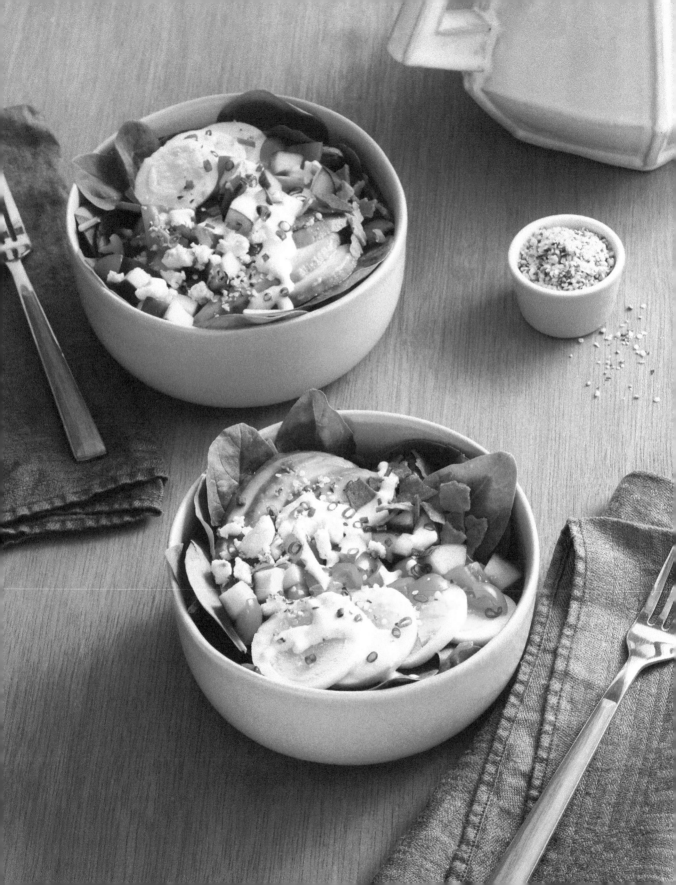

CHAPTER FIVE

Salads, Soups, and Sandwiches

Curried Egg Salad 52

Avocado Egg Salad 53

Classic Creamy Coleslaw 54

Spinach Avocado Salad 55

Greek Cottage Cheese Salad 56

Classic Club Salad 57

▶ Hemp Cobb Salad 58

Mediterranean Salad 59

Avocado and Asparagus Salad 60

Thai Noodle Salad 61

Roasted Cauliflower Lettuce Cups 62

Taco Lettuce Cups 63

Avocado Pesto Panini 64

Loaded Bell Pepper Sandwich 65

Ultimate Grilled Cheese 66

Slow Cooker Broccoli Cheese Soup 67

Instant Pot French Onion Soup 68

Creamed Cauliflower Soup 69

Portobello Mushroom Burger with Avocado 70

CURRIED EGG SALAD

DAIRY-FREE, GLUTEN-FREE
Serves 4 / Prep time: 5 minutes

Eggs are a great source of protein and nutrients for vegetarians on the keto-genic diet. Egg yolks contain HDL fats, which are the good fats, and also high levels of omega-3 fatty acids. For a variation on this tasty recipe, see Avocado Egg Salad (page 53).

6 hardboiled eggs, finely chopped

1 celery stalk, diced

½ cup cashews, finely diced

¼ cup olive oil mayonnaise

1 tablespoon Dijon mustard

1½ teaspoons curry powder

¼ teaspoon salt

¼ teaspoon freshly ground black pepper

8 butter lettuce leaves

1. In a medium mixing bowl, combine the eggs with the celery and cashews.

2. Add the mayonnaise, mustard, curry powder, salt, and pepper, and stir until thoroughly combined.

3. Divide the salad into four equal servings and serve on top of the butter lettuce leaves.

Ingredient tip: Don't have time to boil eggs? Many grocery stores offer ready-to-eat hardboiled eggs.

Per Serving **Calories:** 600; Fat: 50g; Protein: 23g; Total carbs: 15g; Net carbs: 13g; Fiber: 2g; Sugar: 3g; Sodium: 728mg **Macros:** Fat: 75%; Protein: 15%; Carbs: 10%

AVOCADO EGG SALAD

DAIRY-FREE, GLUTEN-FREE, NUT-FREE
Serves 2 / Prep time: 5 minutes

½ avocado, mashed

1 tablespoon freshly squeezed lemon juice

¼ teaspoon salt

¼ teaspoon freshly ground black pepper

6 hardboiled eggs, finely chopped

2 radishes, sliced

1. In a medium bowl, combine the avocado with the lemon juice, salt, and pepper.

2. Add the chopped eggs to the avocado mixture and stir gently to combine.

3. Serve topped with the radish slices.

Per Serving **Calories:** 272; Fat: 20g; Protein: 18g; Total carbs: 5g; Net carbs: 2g; Fiber: 3g; Sugar: 1g; Sodium: 482mg **Macros:** Fat: 66%; Protein: 26%; Carbs: 8%

CLASSIC CREAMY COLESLAW

DAIRY-FREE, EGG-FREE, NUT-FREE
Serves 1 / Prep time: 5 minutes

Vegans and vegetarians often use seitan because it mimics the texture of meat. It comes unflavored but readily absorbs any seasoning you might like to add. It's derived from vital wheat gluten and can be found in most grocery stores.

3 tablespoons veganaise

½ tablespoon white vinegar

3 drops liquid stevia

¼ teaspoon dry mustard

¼ teaspoon salt

¼ teaspoon freshly ground black pepper

1 cup prepared coleslaw mix

3½ ounces seitan strips

1. In a small bowl, stir together the veganaise, vinegar, stevia, mustard, salt, and pepper until well combined.

2. Add the coleslaw mix and fold it in gently.

3. Top with the seitan and add more pepper, if needed.

Change it up: If seitan isn't your thing, try replacing it with ½ avocado, diced.

Per Serving **Calories:** 381; Fat: 29g; Protein: 22g; Total carbs: 8g; Net carbs: 5g; Fiber: 3g; Sugar: 2g; Sodium: 1288mg **Macros:** Fat: 69%; Protein: 23%; Carbs: 8%

SPINACH AVOCADO SALAD

DAIRY-FREE, GLUTEN-FREE, NUT-FREE
Serves 2 / Prep time: 10 minutes

The three most important things to remember for making a great salad: You need to add flavor, there must be some crunch, and, finally, don't waste your time with iceberg lettuce. Get creative, have fun, and don't be scared to try new combinations.

1½ cups fresh spinach leaves

4 hardboiled eggs, chopped

¼ cup chopped carrots

¼ cup chopped cucumbers

½ avocado, sliced

¼ cup diced tomatoes

1 tablespoon olive oil

1 tablespoon balsamic vinegar

Salt

Freshly ground black pepper

1. Place the spinach in a serving dish.

2. Top with the eggs, carrots, cucumbers, avocado, and tomatoes.

3. In a small bowl, mix together the oil and vinegar.

4. Pour the dressing on the salad and season with salt and pepper as needed.

Change it up: If you like more of a crunch, the avocado can be swapped out for some toasted cashews or sunflower seeds.

Per Serving **Calories:** 291; Fat: 23g; Protein: 13g; Total carbs: 8g; Net carbs: 4g; Fiber: 4g; Sugar: 2g; Sodium: 233mg **Macros:** Fat: 71%; Protein: 18%; Carbs: 11%

GREEK COTTAGE CHEESE SALAD

EGG-FREE, GLUTEN-FREE, NUT-FREE
Serves 1 / Prep time: 5 minutes

Cottage cheese is an excellent source of protein for meat-free eaters, and it can also fit right into a vegetarian ketogenic diet. This salad is easy to assemble with just a few ingredients that you may already have in your kitchen.

1 cup 4-percent cottage cheese

⅓ cup halved cherry tomatoes

1 tablespoon chopped scallion, white
   part only

⅓ cup peeled and diced cucumber

2 tablespoons olive oil

½ cup Kalamata olives

Salt

Freshly ground black pepper

In a serving bowl, mix together the cottage cheese, cherry tomatoes, scallion, cucumber, olive oil, and olives, and season with salt and pepper as needed.

Ingredient tip: If you don't have cottage cheese on hand, plain Greek yogurt makes an excellent substitute.

Per Serving **Calories:** 610; Fat: 51g; Protein: 27g; Total carbs: 15g; Net carbs: 11g; Fiber: 4g; Sugar: 9g; Sodium: 1955mg **Macros:** Fat: 72%; Protein: 19%; Carbs: 9%

CLASSIC CLUB SALAD

GLUTEN-FREE, NUT-FREE
Serves 4 / Prep time: 10 minutes

Inspired by the flavors of the famous club sandwich, this salad combines the refreshing flavors of cucumber and tomato with the fat and protein provided by egg and cheese. A decadent creamy dressing ties it all together.

3 tablespoons sour cream

3 tablespoons veganaise

¾ teaspoon garlic powder

¾ teaspoon onion powder

1 teaspoon dried parsley

1 tablespoon heavy (whipping) cream

4 cups coarsely chopped romaine lettuce

1 cup diced cucumber

½ cup halved cherry tomatoes

4 hardboiled eggs, chopped

4 ounces cheddar cheese, grated

1. In a small bowl, mix together the sour cream, veganaise, garlic powder, onion powder, and parsley.

2. Stir in the cream and set aside.

3. Build the salad by layering the lettuce, cucumber, tomatoes, eggs, and cheddar cheese.

4. Divide the salad into 4 servings and top with dressing.

Prep tip: Washing, drying, and cutting lettuce and placing it in a gallon-size resealable bag for storage as soon as you get home allows you to create salads in a matter of minutes.

Per Serving **Calories:** 293; Fat: 24g; Protein: 14g; Total carbs: 5g; Net carbs: 4g; Fiber: 1g; Sugar: 2g; Sodium: 312mg **Macros:** Fat: 74%; Protein: 19%; Carbs: 7%

HEMP COBB SALAD

GLUTEN-FREE, NUT-FREE
Serves 2 / Prep time: 10 minutes

Cobb salads are a staple for keto eaters, and in this rendition, you'll get your salty crunch from vegan bacon. This super fresh, veggie-loaded salad can be easily prepared in just a few minutes.

2 cups fresh spinach leaves

4 hardboiled eggs, chopped

¼ cup diced cucumber

1 avocado, sliced

¼ cup diced tomato

4 slices cooked vegan bacon, sliced

4 tablespoons hemp seeds

2 tablespoons diced scallions, white and green parts

4 tablespoons blue cheese

4 ounces blue cheese dressing

1. Divide the spinach leaves between two bowls.

2. Arrange half the eggs, cucumber, avocado, tomato, and bacon in sections on top of each bowl of spinach.

3. Sprinkle each salad with half the hemp seeds, scallions, and blue cheese.

4. Top each salad with the dressing and serve.

Leftover tip: To store this salad for future use, prepare the ingredients and keep them in separate sandwich bags in the refrigerator for up to three days.

Per Serving **Calories:** 858; Fat: 72g; Protein: 32g; Total carbs: 20g; Net carbs: 11g; Fiber: 9g; Sugar: 4g; Sodium: 1242mg **Macros:** Fat: 76%; Protein: 15%; Carbs: 9%

MEDITERRANEAN SALAD

EGG-FREE, GLUTEN-FREE, NUT-FREE
Servings 2 / Prep time: 10 minutes

This light and fresh salad is bursting with Mediterranean flavors. The Mediterranean diet has long been touted as one of the healthiest diets to follow, mostly due to its emphasis on fresh vegetables and healthy fats. Consuming a good amount of healthy fat in your diet may help prevent Alzheimer's disease as well as boost brain power.

3 tablespoons olive oil

2 tablespoons red wine vinegar

3 garlic cloves, minced

½ teaspoon salt

¼ teaspoon freshly ground black pepper

1 head romaine lettuce, leaves torn into
    small pieces

½ red onion, sliced

½ cup diced cucumber

24 Kalamata olives

2 small Campari tomatoes, diced
    and seeded

1 cup crumbled feta cheese

1. In a small bowl, mix together the olive oil, vinegar, garlic, salt, and pepper. Set aside.

2. In a large bowl, combine the lettuce, onion, cucumber, olives, tomatoes, and feta cheese.

3. Pour the dressing over the salad and toss it well to coat the ingredients. Divide equally between two bowls and serve.

Prep tip: The simple but flavorful dressing can be used for many different salads. You can triple the batch and store it, covered, in the refrigerator for up to 1 week.

Per Serving **Calories:** 515; Fat: 43g; Protein: 13g; Total carbs: 19g; Net carbs: 15g;
Fiber: 4g; Sugar: 8g; Sodium: 1794mg **Macros:** Fat: 75%; Protein: 10%; Carbs: 15%

AVOCADO AND ASPARAGUS SALAD

EGG-FREE, GLUTEN-FREE, NUT-FREE
Serves 4 / Prep time: 15 minutes / Cook time: 2 minutes

The star of this hearty salad combination is super-healthy blanched aspar-agus. Blanching is a simple process that begins with a brief scalding of the vegetable followed by an ice bath. This helps "precook" the vegetable while keeping its nutritional value intact.

½ pound asparagus, trimmed and halved

4 cups red leaf lettuce

1 cup cherry tomatoes, halved

1 ripe avocado, sliced

1 cup sliced mozzarella

¼ cup fresh basil leaves

⅓ cup olive oil

1 teaspoon freshly squeezed lemon juice

½ teaspoon Dijon mustard

Salt

Freshly ground black pepper

1. Prepare an ice bath by filling a large bowl with cold water and plenty of ice.

2. Put a pot of water over medium-high heat and bring to a boil. Add the asparagus to the boiling water and cook for 1 to 2 minutes.

3. Immediately drain the asparagus and transfer it to the ice bath to stop the cooking process. Let cool for 5 minutes.

4. Drain the asparagus and pat it dry with paper towels.

5. Layer equal amounts of lettuce, asparagus, tomatoes, avocado, mozzarella, and basil leaves on four serving plates.

6. In a small bowl, combine the olive oil, lemon juice, and Dijon mustard and add salt and pepper as needed.

7. Pour the dressing evenly over the salads and serve.

Ingredient tip: Dijon mustard can be used for extra flavor in any keto recipe. It is low in calories and carbs, so in terms of the keto diet, it is considered a low-impact food item.

Per Serving (makes 4 servings) **Calories:** 346; Fat: 30g; Protein: 10g; Total carbs: 9g; Net carbs: 4g; Fiber: 5g; Sugar: 3g; Sodium: 235mg **Macros:** Fat: 78%; Protein: 12%; Carbs: 10%

THAI NOODLE SALAD

GLUTEN-FREE, DAIRY-FREE, EGG-FREE
Serves 4 / Prep time: 10 minutes

Shirataki noodles are a keto-friendly alternative to starchy noodles. These noodles can be found in most health food stores or online. They consist primarily of water and fiber and contain traces of protein and fat. The high fiber content will help you feel full and can aid in weight loss. In this recipe, the noodles are paired with cashews and plenty of cruciferous vegetables.

1 cup shredded purple cabbage

1 cup shredded green cabbage

¼ cup chopped scallions

¼ cup chopped fresh cilantro

3 cups shirataki noodles, rinsed and drained

½ cup chopped cashews

2 tablespoons minced garlic

2 tablespoons minced fresh ginger

½ cup water

1 tablespoon freshly squeezed lime juice

1 tablespoon soy sauce

1 tablespoon coconut aminos

⅓ cup creamy natural cashew butter

½ teaspoon salt

Liquid stevia

1. In a large bowl, combine the purple and green cabbage, scallions, cilantro, noodles, and cashews.

2. In a medium bowl, combine the garlic, ginger, water, lime juice, soy sauce, coconut aminos, cashew butter, and salt. Sweeten with stevia as desired. Mix well with a whisk until thoroughly combined.

3. Pour the dressing over the vegetable and noodle mixture, then toss well.

4. Divide into 4 equal servings.

Ingredient tip: Most nuts and nut butters are fairly interchangeable, so if you don't have a particular nut or nut butter called for in a recipe, simply use what you have.

Per Serving **Calories:** 295; Fat: 19g; Protein: 8g; Total carbs: 23g; Net carbs: 17g; Fiber: 6g; Sugar: 4g; Sodium: 532mg **Macros:** Fat: 58%; Protein: 11%; Carbs: 31%

ROASTED CAULIFLOWER LETTUCE CUPS

EGG-FREE, DAIRY-FREE, GLUTEN-FREE
Serves 4 / Prep time: 10 minutes / Cook time: 20 minutes

The trick to keeping your diet exciting as a vegetarian eater is using various cooking methods to add flavor and depth to your vegetables. Roasting vegetables, especially cauliflower, is a great technique because it allows the natural flavors to caramelize and develop a unique taste.

Nonstick cooking spray

1 head cauliflower, chopped

1 tablespoon avocado oil

½ teaspoon minced garlic

2 tablespoons curry powder

½ teaspoon salt

¼ teaspoon freshly ground black pepper

4 butter lettuce leaves

2 avocados, sliced

4 tablespoons cashews

4 tablespoons ranch dressing

1. Preheat the oven to 425°F.

2. Grease a rimmed baking sheet with cooking spray and put the cauliflower florets on it.

3. Pour the avocado oil on the florets and toss to coat; then sprinkle the florets with the garlic, curry powder, salt, and pepper.

4. Roast for about 20 minutes, or until the tops of the florets are slightly browned.

5. Remove from the oven and allow to cool for 5 to 7 minutes.

6. Place a scoop of florets into each butter lettuce cup and top each with ¼ of the avocado slices.

7. Sprinkle each cup with 1 tablespoon of cashews and 1 tablespoon of ranch dressing.

Leftover tip: Roasted vegetables do not keep well in the refrigerator for more than 1 day. If you find yourself with leftover cauliflower, throw it into some scrambled eggs for a quick and easy keto meal.

Per Serving **Calories:** 349; Fat: 29g; Protein: 5g; Total carbs: 17g; Net carbs: 8g; Fiber: 9g; Sugar: 3g; Sodium: 446mg **Macros:** Fat: 75%; Protein: 6%; Carbs: 19%

TACO LETTUCE CUPS

EGG-FREE, GLUTEN-FREE

Serves 4 / Prep time: 10 minutes / Cook time: 5 minutes

Meat substitutes have come a long way in the last few years. If you are new to meat substitutes, these tacos are a great way to learn about them. Most soy-based products are made with GMO soy, so pay attention to the package labels before purchasing. BOCA is a non-GMO brand, which makes it a good choice for these tasty tacos.

2 cups meatless crumbles

1 tablespoon coconut oil

1 cup chopped onion

1 bell pepper, chopped

1½ teaspoons minced garlic

½ pound mushrooms, sliced

1 head butter lettuce, leaves removed

¼ cup chopped fresh cilantro

½ cup salsa

1 cup shredded cheddar cheese

1 avocado, diced

1. In a medium skillet over medium heat, cook the crumbles until thoroughly warmed. Remove them from the skillet and set aside.

2. In the same skillet, melt the coconut oil and sauté the onion, bell pepper, garlic, and mushrooms for 4 to 5 minutes. Remove from the heat and stir in the crumbles.

3. Divide the mixture equally between lettuce cups on four dishes.

4. Top the cups with the cilantro, salsa, cheddar cheese, and avocado.

Ingredient Tip: If butter lettuce isn't readily available, use romaine or kale instead. They are both hearty leaves that can hold the taco filling.

Per Serving **Calories:** 370; Fat: 22g; Protein: 23g; Total carbs: 20g; Net carbs: 14g; Fiber: 6g; Sugar: 6g; Sodium: 584mg **Macros:** Fat: 54%; Protein: 25%; Carbs: 21%

AVOCADO PESTO PANINI

EGG-FREE, GLUTEN-FREE

Serves 1 / Prep time: 5 minutes / Cook time: 10 minutes

Made with olive oil, pine nuts, and basil, pesto has loads of flavor and is high in fat and low in carbs. It can be found at just about any grocery store. Added to a grilled cheese sandwich, it makes for the ultimate comfort food.

2 tablespoons grass-fed butter, at room temperature

2 slices Easy Keto Bread (page 143) or store bought

1 tablespoon basil pesto

2 slices Gruyère cheese

½ medium avocado, sliced

1. Heat a small griddle over medium heat.

2. Spread the butter on one side of each slice of bread.

3. Place one piece of bread, butter-side down, on the griddle and then layer the pesto, cheese, and avocado on top.

4. Top the sandwich with the second slice of bread, butter-side up, and gently press down.

5. Allow to cook for 4 to 5 minutes; then flip carefully and cook for an additional 3 to 4 minutes, or until the bread is golden brown.

Change it up: For a lighter option without the avocado, add an additional tablespoon of basil pesto.

Per Serving **Calories:** 824; Fat: 72g; Protein: 29g; Total carbs: 15g; Net carbs: 7g; Fiber: 8g; Sugar: 3g; Sodium: 480mg **Macros:** Fat: 79%; Protein: 14%; Carbs: 7%

LOADED BELL PEPPER SANDWICH

EGG-FREE, GLUTEN-FREE, NUT-FREE
Serves 1 / Prep time: 5 minutes

This is by far one of my favorite vegetarian sandwiches. Your "bread" is the bell pepper shell, and you can fill it with your choice of vegetables, condiments, and cheese. Pickles always add a fun crunch as well.

1 red bell pepper, halved and seeded

½ cup torn iceberg lettuce

1 tablespoon Dijon mustard

1 slice provolone cheese

¼ cup cucumber slices

1 avocado, sliced

2 sandwich pickles

1. Place the red pepper halves, hollow-side up, on a serving plate.

2. Fill one side with the lettuce, and spread the mustard on the other side.

3. Lay the cheese on the mustard side.

4. Next layer the cucumber, avocado, and pickles. Put the bell pepper halves together to form a sandwich. You can use toothpicks to hold it together until you're ready to eat.

Change it up: Making this sandwich with a green, yellow, or orange bell pepper not only changes the flavor, it adds a different pop of color to your plate.

Per Serving **Calories:** 246; Fat: 18g; Protein: 6g; Total carbs: 15g; Net carbs: 8g; Fiber: 7g; Sugar: 4g; Sodium: 511mg **Macros:** Fat: 66%; Protein: 10%; Carbs: 24%

ULTIMATE GRILLED CHEESE

GLUTEN-FREE

Serves 1 / Prep time: 5 minutes / Cook time: 10 minutes

There's nothing quite like a gooey melted cheese sandwich. Comfort food doesn't get as easy (or as satisfying) as this simple take, which replaces traditional bread with a keto-friendly variety.

1 tablespoon grass-fed butter, at room temperature

2 slices Easy Keto Bread (page 143) or store bought

2 slices cheddar cheese

1. Heat a skillet over medium-high heat.

2. Spread the butter on one side of each slice of bread.

3. Place one slice, butter-side down, in the skillet and top it with the cheddar cheese slices.

4. Top with the second slice of bread, butter-side up, and allow to cook for 4 to 5 minutes.

5. Flip carefully and cook for an additional 3 minutes, or until both sides of bread are golden brown.

6. Remove the sandwich from the skillet and cut in half diagonally.

Change it up: Experimenting with different types of cheeses can add variety to this recipe. The sharper the cheese, the better it will melt.

Per Serving **Calories:** 528; Fat: 47g; Protein: 23g; Total carbs: 5g; Net carbs: 3g; Fiber: 2g; Sugar: 2g; Sodium: 580mg **Macros:** Fat: 80%; Protein: 17%; Carbs: 3%

SLOW COOKER BROCCOLI CHEESE SOUP

EGG-FREE, GLUTEN-FREE, NUT-FREE
Serves 10 / Prep time: 10 minutes / Cook time: 3 hours

Cooking a large batch of soup can be a huge time-saver in the kitchen, and with this recipe, you can set it to cook in the morning and come home to find your meal ready, with enough to set aside for future meals. This broccoli cheese soup has plenty of fiber from the broccoli and healthy fats from the cheeses.

2 cups water

2 cups vegetable broth

8 ounces Greek yogurt cream cheese, at room temperature

1 cup heavy (whipping) cream

2 tablespoons grass-fed butter

5 cups frozen broccoli florets

½ cup Parmesan cheese

2 cups cheddar cheese

½ teaspoon salt

½ teaspoon freshly ground black pepper

1. Turn the slow cooker to high.

2. Combine the water, vegetable broth, cream cheese, heavy cream, and butter in the bowl of the slow cooker and mix well.

3. Add the broccoli and Parmesan cheese, then stir to mix all the ingredients together.

4. Cover the slow cooker and cook for 3 hours.

5. When the cooking time is up, uncover the bowl and sprinkle the soup with the cheddar cheese. Stir until it melts.

6. Add the salt and pepper and serve.

Prep tip: If you don't have access to a slow cooker, you can easily make this soup on the stovetop in a large stockpot over medium heat. Cook, covered, for 20 minutes, stirring occasionally. Then follow steps 5 and 6 as written.

Per Serving (1 cup) **Calories:** 288; Fat: 24g; Protein: 12g; Total carbs: 6g; Net carbs: 5g; Fiber: 1g; Sugar: 1g; Sodium: 507mg **Macros:** Fat: 75%; Protein: 17%; Carbs: 8%

INSTANT POT FRENCH ONION SOUP

EGG-FREE, GLUTEN-FREE, NUT-FREE
Serves 6 / Prep time: 10 minutes / Cook time: 30 minutes

It's hard to imagine that something as decadent as French onion soup can be part of a weight-loss process. But the ketogenic diet allows for foods that are off-limits in other diets due to their high fat content. This rich, delicious soup will quickly become part of your weekly rotation.

1 tablespoon grass-fed butter

2 large white onions, sliced

6 cups vegetable broth

1 tablespoon minced garlic

½ teaspoon salt

1 bay leaf

2 cups shredded Gruyère cheese

1. Turn the Instant Pot to sauté mode and melt the butter. Add the onions and allow them to cook until translucent, 4 to 5 minutes.

2. Pour in the broth, garlic, salt, and bay leaf.

3. Cover the pot with its lid (until it clicks closed), and turn the pot to manual pressure for 25 minutes.

4. Once the timer goes off, turn the Instant Pot off and allow it to natural-release for 10 to 15 minutes. Then release any additional pressure. Divide the soup between six bowls.

5. Sprinkle the cheese on each bowl of soup and serve hot.

Prep tip: To prepare this soup on the stovetop, in a large stockpot on medium heat, melt the butter and sauté the onions until translucent, 4 to 5 minutes. Mix in the broth, garlic, salt, and bay leaf. Bring the soup to a simmer and cook for 20 to 25 minutes, or until the onions are very soft. Divide into 6 servings and sprinkle with the cheese.

Per Serving (1 cup) **Calories:** 222; Fat: 14g; Protein: 16g; Total carbs: 8g; Net carbs: 7g; Fiber: 1g; Sugar: 3g; Sodium: 1045mg **Macros:** Fat: 57%; Protein: 29%; Carbs: 14%

CREAMED CAULIFLOWER SOUP

EGG-FREE, GLUTEN-FREE, NUT-FREE
Serves 4 / Prep time: 10 minutes / Cook time: 30 minutes

Cauliflower is a wonderful keto vegetable. It's low in carbs and high in fiber and can happily take on many different flavors. This thick and creamy cauliflower soup keeps your body in fat-burning mode.

2 tablespoons grass-fed butter

1 white onion, chopped

1 tablespoon minced fresh garlic

1 medium cauliflower, chopped into
  small florets

2 cups vegetable broth

1 bay leaf

1 cup grated sharp cheddar cheese

½ cup heavy (whipping) cream

1 teaspoon salt

½ teaspoon freshly ground black pepper

1. In a stockpot over medium-high heat, melt the butter.

2. Add the onion and garlic and sauté for about 3 minutes.

3. Add the cauliflower florets and cook, stirring, for another 2 to 3 minutes.

4. Pour in the vegetable broth and add the bay leaf.

5. Bring to a simmer and cook for about 20 minutes, or until the cauliflower is tender.

6. Remove from the heat and stir in the cheddar cheese, cream, salt, and pepper. Stir until the cheese is totally melted.

7. Divide into 4 portions and serve.

Prep Tip: To cook this soup in an Instant Pot, turn the pot to sauté and melt the butter. Add the onion and garlic and sauté for 3 minutes. Add the cauliflower and sauté for another 2 minutes or so. Add the broth and bay leaf. Turn the pot to manual pressure for 10 minutes. Allow to natural-release for 10 minutes; then release any remaining pressure, remove the lid, and stir in the cheese, cream, salt, and pepper.

Per Serving **Calories:** 351; Fat: 27g; Protein: 14g; Total carbs: 13g; Net carbs: 9g; Fiber: 4g; Sugar: 5g; Sodium: 1236mg **Macros:** Fat: 69%; Protein: 16%; Carbs: 15%

PORTOBELLO MUSHROOM BURGER WITH AVOCADO

NUT-FREE, GLUTEN-FREE, EGG-FREE
Serves 1 / Prep time: 15 minutes / Cook time: 10 minutes

Yes, you can eat a burger on a vegetarian ketogenic diet. The meaty mushrooms, which are high in niacin, B_6, and B_3—all vital for anyone eating a vegetarian diet—serve as both bun and "beef." The avocado and sprouts smashed between the buns add fat and a ton of beneficial nutrients.

Nonstick cooking spray

4 large portobello mushrooms, destemmed and wiped clean

1 tablespoon avocado oil

½ teaspoon salt

¼ teaspoon freshly ground black pepper

1 avocado, mashed

1 tablespoon full-fat plain Greek yogurt

1 tablespoon veganaise or mayonnaise

1 tablespoon freshly squeezed lime juice

¼ teaspoon ground cumin

½ cup broccoli sprouts

1. Preheat the oven to 400°F. Spray a baking sheet with cooking spray.

2. Brush the tops of the mushrooms with the avocado oil. Place them on the prepared baking sheet (tops up) and sprinkle with the salt and pepper.

3. Cook for 8 to 10 minutes and then flip the mushrooms over and cook for an additional 8 to 10 minutes. Remove from the oven.

4. In a small bowl, combine the avocado, Greek yogurt, veganaise, lime juice, and cumin. Stir together until well blended.

5. Layer half of the avocado mixture between 2 mushroom "buns" and top with half the broccoli sprouts. Repeat to make the second burger.

Ingredient tip: If you are having trouble finding broccoli sprouts, you can swap them for alfalfa or microgreens.

Per Serving (2 burgers) **Calories:** 638; Fat: 50g; Protein: 13g; Total carbs: 34g; Net carbs: 17g; Fiber: 17g; Sugar: 2g; Sodium: 1121mg **Macros:** Fat: 71%; Protein: 8%; Carbs: 21%

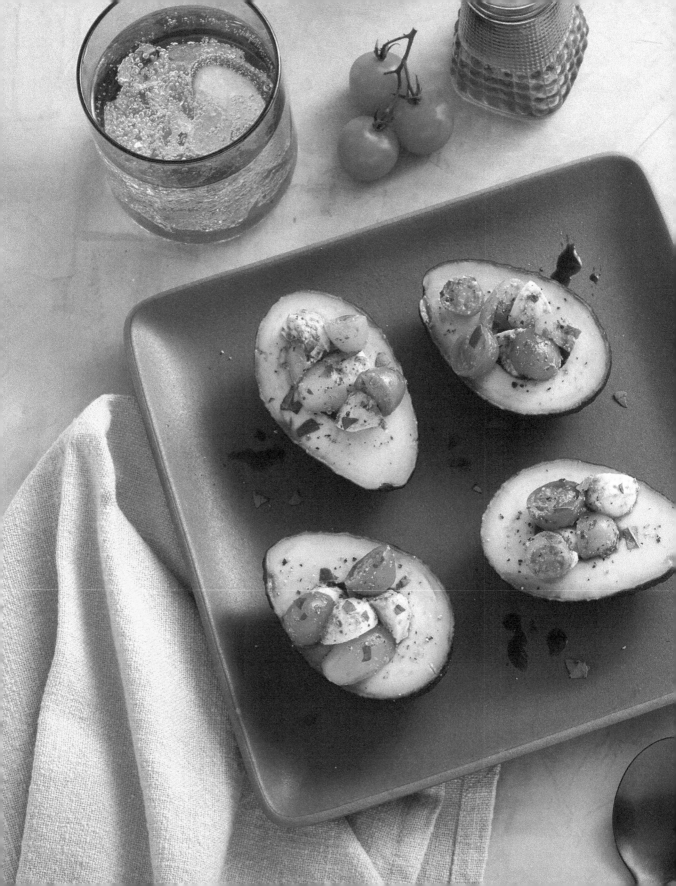

CHAPTER SIX

Snacks, Appetizers, and Savory Fat Bombs

Smoked Almonds 74

Roasted Garlic Mushrooms 75

Mediterranean Cucumber Bites 76

Roasted Cauliflower Hummus 77

Creamy Spinach Dip 78

Parmesan Zucchini Chips 79

Flaxseed Chips and Guacamole 80

Cheesy Crackers 81

▶ Caprese Stuffed Avocados 82

Cheesy Cauliflower Breadsticks 83

Herbed Mozzarella Sticks 85

Baked Olives 86

Zucchini Fritters 87

Three-Cheese Stuffed Mushrooms 88

Savory Party Mix 89

No-Fail Deviled Eggs 90

"Everything but the Bagel" Fat Bombs 91

Cheesy Dill Fat Bombs 92

SMOKED ALMONDS

EGG-FREE, GLUTEN-FREE
Serves 10 / Prep time: 5 minutes / Cook time: 45 minutes

Thanks to a hormone called ghrelin, which stimulates appetite, sometimes we just can't seem to feel full, no matter how well we plan our meals. For those days, try these smoked almonds, which may be one of the best-tasting snacks around. This recipe makes a batch big enough for a crowd or for lots of leftovers.

1 pound raw almonds

2 tablespoons grass-fed butter, melted

2 tablespoons liquid smoke

2 tablespoons Worcestershire sauce

1 tablespoon salt

1. Preheat the oven to 200°F. Line a baking dish with aluminum foil.

2. Put the almonds in a large mixing bowl and set aside.

3. In a small bowl, mix together the butter, liquid smoke, and Worcestershire sauce.

4. Pour the mixture over the almonds and stir. Sprinkle in the salt and mix again.

5. Spread the almonds evenly on the prepared baking dish and place in the oven.

6. Cook for 45 minutes, stirring well every 10 minutes.

7. Once cooked, transfer the nuts to paper towels to drain. When cool, store in an airtight container until ready to serve.

Ingredient tip: These almonds can be used for more than just a snack. Try topping your salads with them for a little bit of crunch and a whole lot of flavor.

Per Serving (about 27) **Calories:** 305; Fat: 25g; Protein: 10g; Total carbs: 10g; Net carbs: 4g; Fiber: 6g; Sugar: 3g; Sodium: 731mg **Macros:** Fat: 74%; Protein: 13%; Carbs: 13%

ROASTED GARLIC MUSHROOMS

EGG-FREE, GLUTEN-FREE, NUT-FREE

Serves 4 / Prep time: 5 minutes / Cook time: 25 minutes

Mushrooms are a popular ingredient in many vegetarian dishes. They add flavor and a hearty texture that is reminiscent of meat. In this recipe, mushrooms are combined with some healthy fat (avocado oil) and flavor (garlic) to create a savory snack.

Nonstick cooking spray

1⅓ pounds cremini mushrooms

6 garlic cloves, minced

3 tablespoons avocado oil

3 tablespoons Parmesan cheese

½ teaspoon salt

¼ teaspoon freshly ground black pepper

3 tablespoons dried parsley

1. Preheat the oven to 400°F. Line a baking sheet with aluminum foil and spray with nonstick cooking spray.

2. In a mixing bowl, combine the mushrooms, garlic, avocado oil, Parmesan cheese, salt, and pepper. Mix well.

3. Spread the mushroom mixture on the prepared baking sheet and sprinkle with the parsley.

4. Bake for 12 minutes and stir. Return to the oven and bake for an additional 12 minutes.

5. Transfer the mushrooms to a serving dish.

Change it up: Experiment with mushroom varieties for different textures and flavors; shiitakes take well to roasting.

Per Serving (⅓ cup) **Calories:** 180; Fat: 13g; Protein: 8g; Total carbs: 8g; Net carbs: 7g; Fiber: 1g; Sugar: 3g; Sodium: 400mg **Macros:** Fat: 66%; Protein: 17%; Carbs: 17%

MEDITERRANEAN CUCUMBER BITES

EGG-FREE, GLUTEN-FREE, NUT-FREE
Serves 4 / Prep time: 10 minutes

These cucumber bites are perfect for hot days when you don't want to turn on the oven. They are simple and easy to make, and you can experiment with different spices to see how they change the flavor. Make sure to keep the cream cheese full fat to keep you in fat-burning keto mode.

8 ounces cream cheese, at room
  temperature
2 tablespoons chopped flat-leaf parsley
⅓ cup diced black olives

1 bell pepper, diced
2 cucumbers, halved lengthwise and seeded
2 tablespoons sliced scallions

1. In a small bowl, mix together the cream cheese, parsley, olives, and bell pepper.

2. Fill each cucumber cavity with the cream cheese mixture. Sprinkle with the scallions, slice into 1-inch pieces, and serve.

Leftovers tip: To store, wrap each filled cucumber tightly in plastic wrap and place in the refrigerator for up to 2 days.

Per Serving (½ cucumber) **Calories:** 253; Fat: 21g; Protein: 6g; Total carbs: 10g; Net carbs: 8g; Fiber: 2g; Sugar: 4g; Sodium: 271mg **Macros:** Fat: 75%; Protein: 9%; Carbs: 16%

ROASTED CAULIFLOWER HUMMUS

DAIRY-FREE, GLUTEN-FREE, NUT-FREE

Serves 6 / Prep time: 20 minutes / Cook time: 40 minutes

Hummus is a close second to edamame when it comes to favorite vegetarian foods. Traditionally a Middle Eastern dish, hummus is widely enjoyed these days. Chickpeas are typically the base for hummus, but here we use the low-carb favorite substitute, cauliflower. Roasting it along with the whole garlic cloves gives the hummus a delicious deep flavor.

Nonstick cooking spray

1 pound cauliflower florets

4 or 5 garlic cloves, peeled but left whole

⅓ cup olive oil

1 tablespoon freshly squeezed lemon juice

½ teaspoon salt

1 teaspoon ground cumin

½ teaspoon paprika

¼ cup water

1. Preheat the oven to 400°F. Line a baking sheet with aluminum foil. Spray with nonstick cooking spray.

2. Place the florets and garlic on the prepared baking sheet. Drizzle with half the olive oil and toss well.

3. Bake for 35 to 40 minutes, or until the vegetables are very tender but not too crispy. Remove from the oven.

4. In a food processor or high-powered blender, combine the florets, garlic, lemon juice, salt, cumin, and paprika. Blend until the mixture forms a smooth purée. While the mixture is blending, pour in the remaining olive oil. Thin out the mixture with water, as needed, until you reach the desired consistency.

5. Transfer the hummus to a bowl and serve.

Pair it with: Choose low-carb, keto-friendly options to serve with this hummus, such as cheesy keto crackers, cucumbers, or celery.

Per Serving **Calories:** 136; Fat: 12g; Protein: 2g; Total carbs: 5g; Net carbs: 3g; Fiber: 2g; Sugar: 2g; Sodium: 218mg **Macros:** Fat: 79%; Protein: 6%; Carbs: 15%

CREAMY SPINACH DIP

EGG-FREE, GLUTEN-FREE, NUT-FREE
Serves 6 / Prep time: 5 minutes / Cook time: 20 minutes

Spinach dip has long been a favorite staple for gatherings. This recipe is similar to a traditional spinach dip, with just a few tweaks for keto. It's simple to make but yields tons of flavor and creaminess, perfect for topping vegetables or even spreading on a piece of keto bread.

Nonstick cooking spray

1 (10-ounce) package frozen spinach, thawed, drained, and squeezed dry

8 ounces cream cheese

8 ounces sour cream

2 tablespoons ranch seasoning

½ cup grated Parmesan cheese

1. Preheat the oven to 350°F. Spray an 8-by-8-inch baking dish with nonstick cooking spray. Set aside.

2. In a small bowl, mix together the spinach with the cream cheese and sour cream until well blended. Stir in the ranch seasoning.

3. Spread the mixture in the prepared baking dish and sprinkle with the Parmesan cheese.

4. Bake for 20 minutes, or until the cheese is melted.

Prep tip: If you're planning for a party, this dip can be made ahead and stored in the refrigerator for up to 4 days.

Per Serving **Calories:** 259; Fat: 23g; Protein: 8g; Total carbs: 5g; Net carbs: 4g; Fiber: 1g; Sugar: 0g; Sodium: 368mg **Macros:** Fat: 80%; Protein: 12%; Carbs: 8%

PARMESAN ZUCCHINI CHIPS

EGG-FREE, GLUTEN-FREE, NUT-FREE
Serves 2 / Prep time: 20 minutes / Cook time: 20 minutes

Zucchini is pretty much the perfect vegetable for keto. It pairs well with just about any flavor combination but really lends itself to Parmesan and garlic. The combination of melted salty cheese and crispy zucchini makes for an irresistible snack.

Nonstick cooking spray

2 medium zucchini, cut into ¼-inch coins

½ teaspoon salt

1 cup grated Parmesan cheese

1 teaspoon garlic powder

½ cup low-sugar marinara sauce

1. Preheat the oven to 425°F. Spray a baking sheet with cooking spray.

2. Put the zucchini slices in a medium bowl and sprinkle with the salt. Set aside for 15 minutes.

3. In a separate bowl, combine the Parmesan cheese and garlic powder.

4. Blot the zucchini with a paper towel and place on the prepared baking sheet.

5. Sprinkle each zucchini coin with a generous amount of the cheese mixture.

6. Bake for 15 to 20 minutes, or until the cheese topping is bubbling.

7. Serve with the marinara sauce for dipping.

Prep tip: Try to cut the zucchini as evenly as possible for best results.

Per Serving **Calories:** 249; Fat: 13g; Protein: 21g; Total carbs: 12g; Net carbs: 9g; Fiber: 3g; Sugar: 5g; Sodium: 1201mg **Macros:** Fat: 47%; Protein: 34%; Carbs: 19%

FLAXSEED CHIPS AND GUACAMOLE

DAIRY-FREE, EGG-FREE, GLUTEN-FREE, NUT-FREE
Serves 6 / Prep time: 10 minutes / Cook time: 60 minutes

Chips and salsa are one of the most commonly requested "cheat meal" foods for those on a strict diet. Luckily, they can be easily made and adapted for the ketogenic diet. Made with nutrient-dense flaxseed, these chips, along with the healthy fat from the avocado, are the perfect snack for curbing cravings.

1 cup whole flaxseeds	3 large avocados, halved
½ cup vegetable broth	½ cup diced red onion
2 teaspoons garlic powder	1 tablespoon freshly squeezed lime juice
2 teaspoons paprika	½ teaspoon salt
2 teaspoons onion powder	¼ teaspoon ground cumin
1 teaspoon onion salt	

1. Preheat the oven to 325°F. Line a baking sheet with parchment paper.

2. In a large mixing bowl, combine flaxseeds, broth, garlic powder, paprika, onion powder, and onion salt, and mix well.

3. Spread into a thin, even layer on the prepared baking sheet and bake for 55 to 60 minutes.

4. While the chips are baking, mash the avocado in a medium mixing bowl.

5. Mix in the red onion, lime juice, salt, and cumin. Cover the bowl and place it in the refrigerator until you are ready to eat.

6. Remove the flaxseed chips from the oven and allow them to cool; then break them apart into chip-size pieces. Serve with the guacamole.

Pair it with: Serve as an appetizer before Mexican Zucchini Hash (page 107) for a filling meal.

Per Serving **Calories:** 328; Fat: 24g; Protein: 8g; Total carbs: 20g; Net carbs: 5g; Fiber: 15g; Sugar: 2g; Sodium: 441mg **Macros:** Fat: 66%; Protein: 10%; Carbs: 24%

CHEESY CRACKERS

GLUTEN-FREE

Makes 55 to 60 crackers / Prep time: 15 minutes / Cook time: 30 minutes

Usually within the first week, a keto eater will miss bread and crackers most of all. These crackers, made with cheese and almond flour, fit the bill as substitutes for white flour–derived foods. They're simple to make and can help curb crunchy, salty cravings!

6 ounces Parmesan cheese

1½ cups almond flour

½ teaspoon salt

½ teaspoon garlic powder

1 egg

2 tablespoons butter, melted

1. Preheat the oven to 300°F. Line a baking sheet with parchment paper.

2. In a medium, microwave-safe bowl, heat the Parmesan cheese in the microwave in 30-second increments until melted, stirring between each cycle.

3. Add the flour, salt, garlic powder, and egg to the cheese mixture. Stir quickly until a dough forms. If the batter seems too sticky, use additional almond flour until it is no longer sticky.

4. Place the dough on a floured surface (or on parchment paper), and roll out to an ⅛-inch thickness. Cut the dough into 1-inch squares and use a spatula to carefully transfer the crackers to the prepared baking sheet.

5. Brush the melted butter across the top of each cracker.

6. Bake the crackers for 25 to 30 minutes, or until the tops are slightly browned.

7. Remove from the oven and allow to cool.

Leftovers tip: These are best stored flat in the pantry in a quart-size, resealable plastic bag.

Per Serving (10 crackers) **Calories:** 256; Fat: 20g; Protein: 14g; Total carbs: 5g; Net carbs: 3g; Fiber: 2g; Sugar: 0g; Sodium: 501mg **Macros:** Fat: 70%; Protein: 22%; Carbs: 8%

CAPRESE STUFFED AVOCADOS

EGG-FREE, GLUTEN-FREE
Serves 4 / Prep time: 10 minutes

Caprese is a popular Italian flavor combination that is usually seen on pizzas and in salads. The main ingredients are tomatoes, mozzarella, basil, and a balsamic glaze or reduction. The word "reduction" often refers to an ingredient in a caramelized state, which would categorize it as non-keto. Here, we use balsamic vinegar because it is much lower in carbs and sugar.

½ cup small mozzarella balls or bocconcini

⅓ cup halved cherry tomatoes

2 tablespoons pesto

2 garlic cloves, minced

1 teaspoon garlic salt

2 avocados, halved

2 tablespoons balsamic vinegar

Freshly ground black pepper

2 tablespoons chopped fresh basil

1. In a medium bowl, mix together the mozzarella, tomatoes, pesto, garlic, and garlic salt.

2. Fill each avocado half with one-fourth of the cheese-and-tomato mixture.

3. Drizzle with the vinegar, season with pepper, and garnish with the basil.

Pair it with: Cheesy Cauliflower Breadsticks (page 83) make a nice, crunchy side for this dish.

Per Serving (1 avocado half) **Calories:** 244; Fat: 20g; Protein: 6g; Total carbs: 10g; Net carbs: 4g; Fiber: 6g; Sugar: 2g; Sodium: 145mg **Macros:** Fat: 74%; Protein: 10%; Carbs: 16%

CHEESY CAULIFLOWER BREADSTICKS

GLUTEN-FREE, NUT-FREE
Serves 6 / Prep time: 25 minutes / Cook time: 35 minutes

The first time you make this recipe, it may seem like a bit of work, but once you become familiar with how a low-carb crust is made, the results will be absolutely worth the time it takes to prepare it. Cauliflower crusts hold up well after cooking and have a neutral flavor that lends itself to a crispy, bread-like crust.

1 head cauliflower, chopped into florets

4 egg whites

½ cup grated sharp cheddar cheese, divided

½ cup grated Parmesan cheese, divided

1 teaspoon dried oregano

¼ teaspoon salt

1. Preheat the oven to 450°F. Line a baking sheet with parchment paper.

2. Put the cauliflower florets in a food processor and pulse until the florets are as small as grains of rice.

3. Transfer the cauliflower to a microwave-safe bowl and cook in the microwave for 7 minutes. Remove and allow to cool for 5 minutes.

4. Pour the cooked cauliflower into a cheesecloth or clean kitchen towel and squeeze to remove as much moisture as possible. The drier the cauliflower, the better the result.

5. In a medium mixing bowl, combine the cauliflower, egg whites, ¼ cup of the cheddar cheese, ¼ cup of Parmesan cheese, oregano, and salt. Mix until a dough forms.

6. Place the dough on top of the parchment paper on the baking sheet. Use a rolling pin to roll it out into a rectangle or circle about ¼ inch thick.

CONTINUED

7. Cook the cauliflower crust for 16 to 18 minutes or until light golden brown.

8. Remove the baking sheet from the oven and top the crust with the remaining ¼ cup of cheddar and ¼ cup of Parmesan cheese. Bake for an additional 5 minutes. Turn the oven to low broil and broil for 3 minutes, or until the cheese is bubbling.

9. Remove from the oven, cut into 12 breadsticks, and serve warm.

Prep tip: Double the batch for the crust. After step 5, wrap the dough ball in plastic wrap and freeze for up to 2 months. Once you are ready to use it, thaw it in the refrigerator for 24 hours and then continue with the recipe as written from step 6.

Per Serving (2 breadsticks) **Calories:** 93; Fat: 5g; Protein: 9g; Total carbs: 3g; Net carbs: 2g; Fiber: 1g; Sugar: 1g; Sodium: 277mg **Macros:** Fat: 48%; Protein: 39%; Carbs: 13%

HERBED MOZZARELLA STICKS

GLUTEN-FREE

Serves 8 / Prep time: 10 minutes / Cook time: 20 minutes

Traditional mozzarella sticks are coated with breadcrumbs, which adds to their carb count. A simple switch enables you to still enjoy these treats: more cheese! Grated almost to a powder, Parmesan is fine enough to coat the mozzarella sticks and crisp up just like breadcrumbs.

½ cup peanut oil

1 cup very finely grated Parmesan cheese

1 tablespoon Italian seasoning

½ teaspoon garlic salt

8 sticks full-fat string cheese, halved horizontally

2 eggs, beaten

1. Pour the peanut oil into a small skillet over high heat. Line a plate with paper towels.

2. While the oil is heating, in a small bowl, mix together the grated Parmesan cheese, Italian seasoning, and garlic salt.

3. Dredge each mozzarella stick first in the beaten egg and then in the cheese-and-herb mixture, rolling the sticks so they are fully coated.

4. Carefully slip 3 or 4 sticks into the hot oil. Cook until all sides are golden brown, about 3 minutes.

5. Transfer to the paper towel–lined plate to drain for a few minutes.

6. Repeat with the remaining cheese sticks, and serve warm.

Per Serving (2 sticks) **Calories:** 425; Fat: 33g; Protein: 28g; Total carbs: 4g; Net carbs: 4g; Fiber: 0g; Sugar: 1g; Sodium: 623mg **Macros:** Fat: 70%; Protein: 26%; Carbs: 4%

BAKED OLIVES

EGG-FREE, GLUTEN-FREE, NUT-FREE
Serves 6 / Prep time: 5 minutes / Cook time: 30 minutes

Olives are technically considered a fruit, and while on keto, the rule is to not eat much fruit. However, olives are an exception to the rule. They are high in fat and low in carbohydrates and contain many micronutrients important to sustaining energy while in ketosis. In this recipe, they are mixed with fresh herbs, feta cheese, and olive oil and baked so they acquire a richer, deeper flavor. Enjoy!

Nonstick cooking spray

1 (6-ounce) can black olives, drained

1 (6-ounce) jar green olives, drained

14 ounces feta cheese, crumbled

2 tablespoons minced fresh rosemary

2 tablespoons minced fresh thyme

2 tablespoons olive oil

1. Preheat the oven to 350°F. Spray an 8-by-8-inch baking dish with cooking spray.

2. Pour the olives into the prepared dish. Stir in the feta cheese, rosemary, and thyme.

3. Drizzle the olive oil on top and mix well until the olives and cheese are well coated.

4. Bake for 22 to 25 minutes. Turn the oven to low broil and broil for an additional 2 to 4 minutes, or until the olives are browned.

5. Remove from the oven and serve warm.

Per Serving **Calories:** 284; Fat: 24g; Protein: 10g; Total carbs: 7g; Net carbs: 5g; Fiber: 2g; Sugar: 3g; Sodium: 1241mg **Macros:** Fat: 76%; Protein: 14%; Carbs: 10%

ZUCCHINI FRITTERS

GLUTEN-FREE

Serves 8 / Prep time: 20 minutes / Cook time: 15 minutes

Zucchini fritters are a savory alternative to pancakes and are popular as a low-carb side dish. The tip for success with these fritters is to make sure that the zucchini is very dry before cooking; otherwise they can become soggy.

2 cups grated zucchini

½ teaspoon salt

2 eggs, beaten

½ teaspoon baking powder

½ cup almond flour

2 tablespoons coconut flour

¼ cup Parmesan cheese

½ cup peanut oil

½ cup sour cream

2 tablespoons chopped fresh chives

1. Line a plate with paper towels.

2. In a medium bowl, sprinkle the zucchini with the salt. Set aside for 5 minutes. Transfer the zucchini to a colander and squeeze it dry with more paper towels.

3. Once the zucchini is as dry as possible, return it to the bowl. Add the eggs, baking powder, almond flour, coconut flour, and Parmesan cheese. Mix until well combined and a batter forms. Set aside.

4. Pour the oil into a small skillet over high heat.

5. Using ¼ cup of batter per fritter, pour batter into the hot skillet and spread into flat pancakes. Cook for 3 minutes, flip, and cook for an additional 3 minutes. Transfer to the paper towel–lined plate to drain.

6. Repeat to make more fritters until all the batter has been used.

7. Serve each fritter topped with 1 tablespoon of sour cream and sprinkled with chives.

Change it up: Topping with full-fat Greek yogurt instead of sour cream adds a different kind of tanginess.

Per Serving (1 fritter) **Calories:** 166; Fat: 14g; Protein: 5g; Total carbs: 5g; Net carbs: 3g; Fiber: 2g; Sugar: 1g; Sodium: 207mg **Macros:** Fat: 76%; Protein: 12%; Carbs: 12%

THREE-CHEESE STUFFED MUSHROOMS

EGG-FREE, GLUTEN-FREE, NUT-FREE
Serves 4 / Prep time: 10 minutes / Cook time: 15 minutes

Stuffed mushrooms are a popular appetizer, one that maybe people don't realize is keto. This recipe is great for preparing ahead of time, so it is perfect for parties. About 20 minutes prior to the party, pop the mushrooms in the oven, and they will be ready right on time. Juicy on the outside, creamy on the inside, and tasty through and through, this dish will satisfy all your guests.

12 button mushrooms, wiped clean and
  stems removed

1 tablespoon olive oil

4 ounces cream cheese

½ cup grated Parmesan cheese

½ cup grated Gruyère cheese

3 garlic cloves, minced

2 tablespoons chopped fresh parsley

¼ teaspoon garlic salt

1. Preheat the oven to 375°F. Line a baking sheet with parchment paper.

2. In a small bowl, toss the mushroom caps with the olive oil. Place the caps upside down on the prepared baking sheet.

3. In a separate small bowl, beat together the cream cheese, Parmesan cheese, Gruyère cheese, garlic, parsley, and garlic salt.

4. Fill each mushroom cap with the cheese mixture.

5. Bake for 15 minutes, and serve warm.

Prep tip: The best way to clean mushrooms is to wipe them with a damp paper towel; submerging them in water can make them soggy.

Per Serving (3 mushrooms) **Calories:** 257; Fat: 21g; Protein: 12g; Total carbs: 5g; Net carbs: 4g; Fiber: 1g; Sugar: 1g; Sodium: 247mg **Macros:** Fat: 74%; Protein: 19%; Carbs: 7%

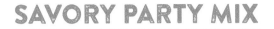

SAVORY PARTY MIX

DAIRY-FREE, EGG-FREE, GLUTEN-FREE
Serves 12 / Prep time: 5 minutes / Cook time: 20 minutes

This party mix is a favorite for parties and gatherings all year long. Party mix is usually made with a rice- or corn-based cereal, but this recipe is tweaked to fit perfectly into a ketogenic diet.

½ cup pecans

½ cup cashews

½ cup pistachios

½ cup peanuts

½ cup almonds

½ cup pumpkin seeds

½ cup sunflower seeds

2 teaspoons onion powder

1 teaspoon garlic powder

½ teaspoon salt

2 tablespoons olive oil

1. Preheat the oven to 350°F. Line a baking sheet with parchment paper.

2. In a large mixing bowl, combine the pecans, cashews, pistachios, peanuts, almonds, pumpkin seeds, and sunflower seeds. Stir in the onion powder, garlic powder, and salt. Pour in the oil. Toss well to thoroughly coat the nuts and seeds with the oil.

3. Spread the mixture in a single layer on the prepared baking sheet and bake for 10 minutes. Stir well and place back in the oven to bake for 10 additional minutes.

4. Remove from the oven and allow to cool completely before serving.

Change it up: Feel free to replace the nuts given here with your favorite kind of nuts; just make sure to keep the quantities the same.

Per Serving (⅓ cup) **Calories:** 214; Fat: 18g; Protein: 6g; Total carbs: 7g; Net carbs: 5g; Fiber: 2g; Sugar: 1g; Sodium: 114mg **Macros:** Fat: 76%; Protein: 11%; Carbs: 13%

NO-FAIL DEVILED EGGS

DAIRY-FREE, GLUTEN-FREE, NUT-FREE
Serves 6 / Prep time: 20 minutes / Cook time: 15 minutes

Deviled eggs are easy to make, loved by nearly everyone, and keto friendly. Make these often, as they are a great snack to keep on hand.

6 hardboiled eggs

3 tablespoons veganaise

3 tablespoons relish

1 teaspoon Dijon mustard

1 teaspoon apple cider vinegar

Paprika

1. Cut each egg in half vertically and scoop out the yolks. Place the yolks in a small bowl.

2. Add the veganaise, relish, mustard, and apple cider vinegar and mash well.

3. Use a spatula to scrape the yolk mixture into a sandwich-size plastic bag, and cut a small triangle off one bottom corner of the bag. Squeeze about 1 tablespoon of yolk mixture into the hollow of each egg-white half.

4. Sprinkle each egg half with paprika.

5. Arrange the eggs on a serving dish and serve immediately.

Prep tip: The following is my favorite method for making perfect hardboiled eggs: Put a pot of water over high heat and bring the water to a boil. Place the eggs in the pot, reduce the heat, and cover. Increase the heat to medium high and boil for 14 minutes. Transfer the eggs to an ice bath until cooled; then peel.

Per Serving (2 eggs) **Calories:** 118; Fat: 9g; Protein: 6g; Total carbs: 3g; Net carbs: 3g; Fiber: 0g; Sugar: 2g; Sodium: 174mg **Macros:** Fat: 67%; Protein: 20%; Carbs: 13%

"EVERYTHING BUT THE BAGEL" FAT BOMBS

EGG-FREE, GLUTEN-FREE, NUT-FREE
Serves 7 / Prep time: 10 minutes, plus 1 hour 30 minutes chill time

It's true that foods and flavors have trends, and right now it seems as though there is nothing hotter than "Everything but the Bagel." This seasoning, a blend of poppy seeds, sesame seeds, dried garlic, dried onion, and salt, is good on just about everything. And if you find yourself craving bread during keto, this recipe will keep you right on track, giving you all the flavors of a savory New York bagel.

8 ounces cream cheese, at room temperature

2 cups shredded cheddar cheese

1 (2.3-ounce) jar "Everything but the Bagel" seasoning

1. In a medium bowl or in a food processor, combine the cream cheese and cheddar cheese until well mixed.

2. Put the mixture in the refrigerator to harden for 1 hour.

3. Line a baking sheet with parchment paper. Pour the seasoning onto a flat plate and set aside.

4. Remove the cheese mixture from the refrigerator and roll it into 1-inch balls. Roll each ball in the seasoning mix until completely covered. Transfer the coated balls to the prepared baking sheet.

5. Place the baking sheet in the refrigerator to chill for 30 mins.

Leftovers tip: Store extra fat bombs in an airtight container (not a plastic bag) so they can retain their shape. They will keep well in the refrigerator for up to 3 days.

Per Serving (2 balls) **Calories:** 246; Fat: 22g; Protein: 11g; Total carbs: 1g; Net carbs: 1g; Fiber: 0g; Sugar: 0g; Sodium: 620mg **Macros:** Fat: 80%; Protein: 19%; Carbs: 1%

CHEESY DILL FAT BOMBS

EGG-FREE, GLUTEN-FREE, NUT-FREE

Serves 7 / Prep time: 10 minutes, plus 1 hour 30 minutes chill time

Fat bombs are a staple in the ketogenic diet because they are high in fat, easy to make, and delicious. Most fat bombs have a cream-cheese base and ingredients added for flavor and texture. This dill creation will help keep any snack cravings at bay while keeping ketones burning high.

8 ounces cream cheese, at room
  temperature

2 cups shredded cheddar cheese

6 mini dill pickles, finely chopped

2 tablespoons minced fresh dill

1. In a medium bowl or in a food processor, combine the cream cheese and cheddar cheese until well mixed.

2. Fold in the pickles and dill.

3. Put the mixture in the refrigerator to harden for 1 hour.

4. Line a baking sheet with parchment paper.

5. Remove the cheese mixture from the refrigerator and roll it into 1-inch balls. Transfer the balls to the prepared baking sheet.

6. Place the baking sheet in the refrigerator to chill for 30 minutes.

Leftovers tip: Store extra fat bombs in an airtight container (not a plastic bag) so they can retain their shape. They will keep well in the refrigerator for up to 3 days.

Per Serving (2 balls) **Calories:** 254; Fat: 22g; Protein: 11g; Total carbs: 3g; Net carbs: 2g; Fiber: 1g; Sugar: 1g; Sodium: 972mg **Macros:** Fat: 78%; Protein: 17%; Carbs: 5%

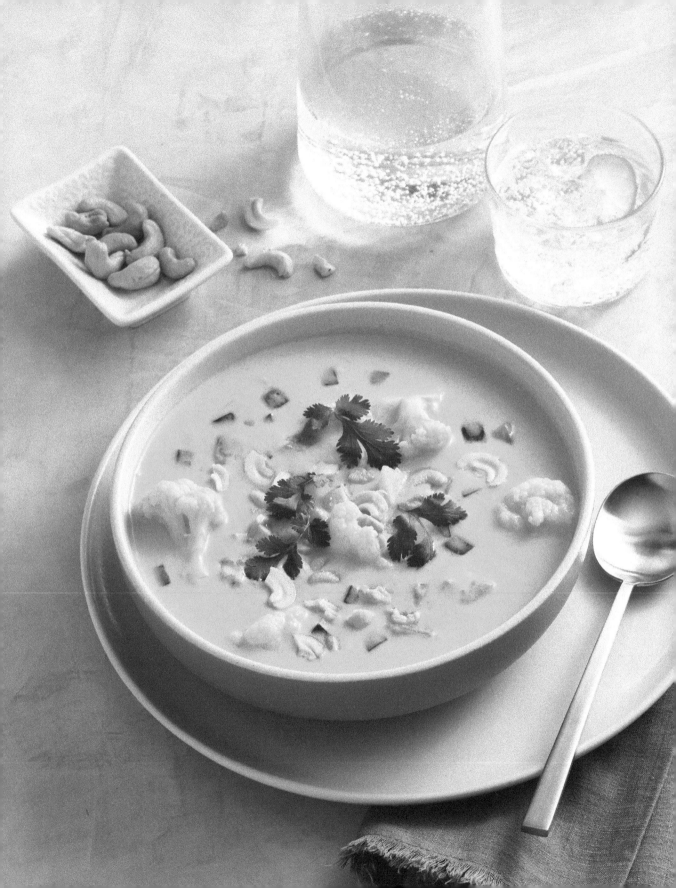

CHAPTER SEVEN

Hearty Main Dishes

Green Goddess Buddha Bowl 96

Zucchini Sage Pasta 97

Broccoli Stir-Fry 98

Kale and Cashew Stir-Fry 99

Tofu Green Bean Casserole 100

Creamy Stuffed Peppers 101

Zucchini Pizza Boats 102

▶ Vegan Coconut Curry 103

Chiles Rellenos 104

Broccoli and Cauliflower Rice Casserole 105

Cauliflower Fried Rice 106

Mexican Zucchini Hash 107

Eggplant Lasagna 108

Spaghetti Squash Bake 109

Cheesy Spinach Bake 110

Fakeachini Alfredo 111

Cheesy Cauliflower Mac 'n' Cheese 112

Margherita Pizza 113

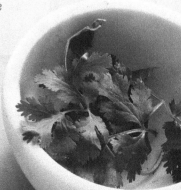

GREEN GODDESS BUDDHA BOWL

DAIRY-FREE, EGG-FREE, GLUTEN-FREE
Serves 1 / Prep time: 10 minutes / Cook time: 5 minutes

Buddha bowls are bowls stuffed with vegetables, fats, and proteins and are a great way to get some delicious nutrition. They often start with a bed of grains, but in this recipe we change it to a bed of fresh spinach to keep it keto. Often, they are topped with a drizzle of flavor such as hummus or tahini, but here it's kept low carb with some savory almond butter.

2 cups fresh spinach

2 tablespoons avocado oil

4 broccolini spears

⅛ teaspoon salt

⅛ teaspoon freshly ground black pepper

⅓ cup frozen cauliflower rice, thawed

2 tablespoons shredded carrots

½ avocado, sliced

1 tablespoon almond butter, melted

1 tablespoon minced fresh cilantro

1. Place the spinach in the bottom of a medium serving bowl.

2. In a skillet over medium-high heat, heat the avocado oil. Add the broccolini and sauté for 2 to 3 minutes. Season with the salt and pepper and transfer it to the bowl containing the spinach.

3. Add the cauliflower rice to the skillet and cook for 3 minutes. Add it to the serving bowl.

4. Top with the carrots and avocado.

5. Drizzle with the melted almond butter, sprinkle the cilantro on top, and serve.

Change it up: Instead of spinach, try kale, chard, red leaf lettuce, or butter lettuce for variety.

Per Serving **Calories:** 571; Fat: 51g; Protein: 9g; Total carbs: 19g; Net carbs: 8g; Fiber: 11g; Sugar: 4g; Sodium: 380mg **Macros:** Fat: 80%; Protein: 6%; Carbs: 14%

ZUCCHINI SAGE PASTA

EGG-FREE, GLUTEN-FREE, NUT-FREE
Serves 1 / Prep time: 10 minutes / Cook time: 5 minutes

Sage is a popular spice for holiday dishes. It is rich in minerals, including potassium, calcium, manganese, and zinc. It has a strong taste, so less is more when cooking with it. This zoodle pasta has a rich, deep flavor and keeps the carbs on the lighter side.

1 tablespoon grass-fed butter

1 tablespoon dried sage

¼ teaspoon ground nutmeg

1 zucchini, spiralized

2 ounces tofu, chopped

1 cup fresh spinach leaves

½ cup grated Parmesan cheese

1. In a skillet over medium-high heat, melt the butter.

2. Add the sage and nutmeg and stir until fragrant, 1 to 2 minutes.

3. Stir in the zucchini and tofu, and cook, stirring, for 3 to 4 minutes.

4. Next, add the spinach and cook for an additional minute until the spinach wilts.

5. Remove from the heat and top with the Parmesan cheese.

6. Serve warm.

Prep tip: To save time, you can buy pre-spiralized bags of zucchini at many grocery stores.

Per Serving **Calories:** 399; Fat: 27g; Protein: 27g; Total carbs: 12g; Net carbs: 8g; Fiber: 4g; Sugar: 4g; Sodium: 659mg **Macros:** Fat: 61%; Protein: 27%; Carbs: 12%

BROCCOLI STIR-FRY

DAIRY-FREE, EGG-FREE, NUT-FREE
Serves 1 / Prep time: 5 minutes / Cook time: 10 minutes

If you are new to vegetarian eating, you may not be familiar with seitan. Seitan is a product made from vital wheat gluten and is high in protein and low in carbs. It has a chewy texture, which makes it a good meat substitute. In this stir-fry, the seitan is paired with green vegetables and healthy fats for a perfect keto dish.

1 cup fresh spinach

1 tablespoon coconut oil

½ cup broccoli florets

1 cup frozen cauliflower rice

2 ounces seitan strips or cubes

1 tablespoon toasted sesame oil

1 tablespoon soy sauce

½ avocado, sliced

1. In a dry, nonstick pan over medium heat, wilt the spinach leaves. Remove from the heat and transfer to a serving plate.

2. Turn the temperature up to medium high, and in the same skillet, melt the coconut oil. Add the broccoli and frozen cauliflower rice. Cook for 5 to 6 minutes or until tender.

3. Place the vegetables on the wilted spinach. Top with the seitan.

4. In a small bowl, mix together the sesame oil and soy sauce.

5. Pour the dressing over the seitan and vegetables. Top with the avocado slices and enjoy warm.

Change it up: To make the dressing soy-free (for allergies or preference), tamari is an excellent alternative to soy sauce.

Per Serving **Calories:** 664; Fat: 44g; Protein: 49g; Total carbs: 18g; Net carbs: 5g; Fiber: 13g; Sugar: 4g; Sodium: 1857mg **Macros:** Fat: 60%; Protein: 30%; Carbs: 10%

KALE AND CASHEW STIR-FRY

DAIRY-FREE, EGG-FREE, GLUTEN-FREE
Serves 1 / Prep time: 5 minutes / Cook time: 5 minutes

Grains might be out of the question on keto, but the good news is that cauliflower rice is an awesome substitute for regular rice. Its recent rise in popularity is due to its versatility and neutral flavor. Cauliflower rice can easily be found in the frozen food section of most grocery stores and is a great keto staple to have on hand.

1 tablespoon coconut oil

1 cup frozen cauliflower rice (or pearls)

½ cup frozen stir-fry vegetables

1 cup destemmed and torn kale
  (small pieces)

3 tablespoons tamari sauce or low-sodium
  soy sauce

⅓ cup chopped cashews

1. In a skillet over medium heat, melt the coconut oil. Add the cauliflower, stir-fry vegetables, and kale, and cook for 2 to 3 minutes, or until tender but still crisp.

2. Pour in the tamari and toss the vegetables until they are coated with the sauce.

3. Transfer the stir-fry to a serving dish, top with the cashews, and enjoy.

Per Serving **Calories:** 523; Fat: 35g; Protein: 18g; Total carbs: 34g; Net carbs: 28g; Fiber: 6g; Sugar: 6g; Sodium: 2173mg **Macros:** Fat: 60%; Protein: 14%; Carbs: 26%

TOFU GREEN BEAN CASSEROLE

EGG-FREE, GLUTEN-FREE, NUT-FREE
Serves 8 / Prep time: 15 minutes / Cook time: 25 minutes

With the ketogenic diet, most green vegetables are considered low impact because they have a high fiber count, which results in a lower net carb number. This green bean casserole will remind you of the one you grew up eating, but with a keto spin, of course. The addition of tofu makes this dish high in protein.

Nonstick cooking spray

1 cauliflower head, chopped into florets

2 tablespoons coconut oil

¼ cup chopped onion

14 ounces green beans, trimmed

1 tablespoon salt

¼ teaspoon freshly ground black pepper

¾ cup full-fat coconut milk

10 ounces tofu

2 cups grated Parmesan cheese

1 cup shredded mozzarella cheese

1. Preheat the oven to 250°F. Grease a 9-by-13-inch casserole dish with cooking spray.

2. Put the cauliflower florets in a microwave-safe dish. Add 1 to 2 tablespoons of water and cover the dish with plastic wrap. Microwave the cauliflower for 8 minutes, or until tender enough to mash.

3. While the cauliflower is cooking, heat a skillet over medium heat and melt the coconut oil. Add the onions and green beans, and cook until slightly tender and bright green.

4. Once the cauliflower is cooked, transfer it to a high-powered blender. Add the salt, pepper, and coconut milk. Pulse until creamy.

5. Spread the cauliflower mash in an even layer in the prepared casserole dish. Place the green beans on top of the mash, and then crumble the tofu on top.

6. Cover with the Parmesan and mozzarella cheeses.

7. Bake the casserole for 15 minutes. For a bubbly cheesy crust, broil the casserole uncovered under a low heat for 1 to 2 minutes.

Leftovers tip: Store any leftovers in individual meal prep containers for a quick grab-and-go option.

Per Serving **Calories:** 297; Fat: 21g; Protein: 18g; Total carbs: 9g; Net carbs: 6g; Fiber: 3g; Sugar: 3g; Sodium: 1231mg **Macros:** Fat: 64%; Protein: 24%; Carbs: 12%

CREAMY STUFFED PEPPERS

GLUTEN-FREE, NUT-FREE
Serves 2 / Prep time: 10 minutes / Cook time: 15 minutes

Bell peppers contain high levels of vitamins A and C, which help increase your body's absorption of iron. They are also high in dietary fiber, which means fewer net carbs. In this recipe, bell peppers take center stage, stuffed with a savory cheese filling.

2 green bell peppers, halved and deseeded

1 tablespoon olive oil

¼ cup chopped onion

1 teaspoon minced garlic

1 cup fresh spinach

12 ounces full-fat ricotta cheese

1 large egg

1 teaspoon dried basil

8 tablespoons grated Parmesan cheese

1. Preheat the oven to 350°F. Line a baking sheet with aluminum foil.

2. Place the bell peppers on the baking sheet, cut-side up, and bake for 10 minutes. Set aside.

3. While the peppers are baking, set a skillet over medium-high heat and pour in the olive oil. Add the onion, garlic, and spinach and sauté for 2 minutes, or until the spinach is wilted.

4. Transfer the mixture to a mixing bowl. Stir in the ricotta cheese, egg, and basil. Mix well.

5. Fill each pepper half with equal amounts of filling and top with 2 tablespoons of Parmesan cheese.

6. Return the peppers to the oven and bake for an additional 5 minutes. Remove and serve.

Change it up: To make this dish egg-free, use a mixture of 1 tablespoon of flaxseed meal and 3 tablespoons of water, refrigerated for 15 minutes or until thickened.

Per Serving (2 pepper halves) **Calories:** 546; Fat: 38g; Protein: 33g; Total carbs: 18g; Net carbs: 15g; Fiber: 3g; Sugar: 7g; Sodium: 457mg **Macros:** Fat: 63%; Protein: 24%; Carbs: 13%

ZUCCHINI PIZZA BOATS

EGG-FREE, GLUTEN-FREE, NUT-FREE
Serves 1 / Prep time: 10 minutes / Cook time: 30 minutes

Zucchini is another versatile vegetable perfect for many ketogenic recipes. In this recipe, the zucchini are hollowed out, leaving the fiber-rich peel and the structure for the pizza boat. The ricotta adds a healthy amount of protein and calcium. This is a recipe you will want on repeat.

1 medium zucchini, halved lengthwise and deseeded

2 tablespoons olive oil

2 garlic cloves, minced

1 cup fresh spinach

2 tablespoons low-sugar marinara sauce

8 ounces full-fat ricotta cheese

1. Line a baking sheet with aluminum foil.

2. Place the zucchini, hollow-side up, on the prepared baking sheet.

3. In a small skillet over medium-high heat, warm the olive oil.

4. Add the garlic and stir for 1 to 2 minutes or until fragrant; then add the spinach and stir until it wilts.

5. Divide the spinach mixture evenly between the zucchini halves. Top evenly with the marinara sauce and ricotta cheese.

6. Bake for 20 to 25 minutes, or until the cheese is melted and the zucchini is tender.

Per Serving **Calories:** 689; Fat: 57g; Protein: 28g; Total carbs: 16g; Net carbs: 14g; Fiber: 3g; Sugar: 4g; Sodium: 251mg **Macros:** Fat: 74%; Protein: 16%; Carbs: 10%

VEGAN COCONUT CURRY

DAIRY-FREE, EGG-FREE, GLUTEN-FREE
Serves 4 / Prep time: 15 minutes / Cook time: 30 minutes

This aromatic curry has a great flavor and will likely make it into your weekly rotation of favorite vegetarian ketogenic meals. Curries are often served with rice or naan, but for keto we can just "beef" up the vegetables a little and enjoy them with some cashews.

2 tablespoons olive oil

½ yellow onion, diced

3 garlic cloves, minced

½ tablespoon minced fresh ginger

1 teaspoon garam masala

1 teaspoon curry powder

1 teaspoon ground cumin

1 (14-ounce) can diced, no-sugar-added tomatoes

3 (14-ounce) cans full-fat coconut milk

1 cauliflower head, cut into florets

2 large zucchini, diced

1 cup chopped cashews

1. In a stockpot over medium-high heat, warm the olive oil. Add the onion and sauté for 2 to 3 minutes.

2. Stir in the garlic, ginger, garam masala, curry powder, cumin, and tomatoes. Cook for 2 minutes.

3. Pour in the coconut milk and bring the mixture to a low simmer. Reduce the heat to low and simmer for 5 minutes. Stir in the cauliflower and zucchini, and simmer for an additional 20 minutes.

4. Top with the chopped cashews and serve.

Change it up: Feel free to switch out veggies as desired, but make sure to stay away from starchy ingredients such as corn or potatoes.

Per Serving **Calories:** 997; Fat: 89g; Protein: 15g; Total carbs: 34g; Net carbs: 22g; Fiber: 12g; Sugar: 18g; Sodium: 91mg **Macros:** Fat: 80%; Protein: 6%; Carbs: 14%

CHILES RELLENOS

EGG-FREE, GLUTEN-FREE, NUT-FREE
Serves 8 / Prep time: 15 minutes / Cook time: 50 minutes

As delicious as Mexican food is, most of it isn't keto. Beans, rice, and tortillas are all way too high in carbs to consider, but luckily one of the favorites on any Mexican takeout menu is the chile relleno. Stuffed with cheese and spinach, these chiles will surely quench any chips-and-salsa cravings.

Nonstick cooking spray

8 poblano chiles

1 tablespoon olive oil

½ onion, chopped

2 garlic cloves, minced

1 cup chopped button mushrooms

4 cups fresh spinach

½ cup sour cream

½ cup heavy (whipping) cream

16 ounces shredded pepper Jack cheese

1. Preheat the oven to 450°F. Spray a baking dish with cooking spray.

2. Cut a slit down the length of each pepper and carefully scoop out and discard all the seeds and membranes. Cut another slit horizontally at the top of the peppers to make an opening for the filling.

3. Place the peppers in the prepared baking dish and cook for about 20 minutes, or until they start to blister. Remove and set aside.

4. While the peppers are in the oven, set a skillet over medium-high heat and pour in the olive oil. Add the onion, garlic, and mushrooms and cook until fragrant, 2 to 3 minutes. Add the spinach and cook until wilted, 4 to 5 minutes.

5. Transfer the mushroom mixture to a medium mixing bowl. Add the sour cream, heavy cream, and pepper Jack cheese, and stir until combined.

6. Remove the peppers from the oven and stuff each one with an equal amount of filling. Close with a toothpick.

7. Return the peppers to the oven for an additional 15 minutes, or until the cheese is melted. Serve warm.

Per Serving (1 pepper) **Calories:** 341; Fat: 29g; Protein: 16g; Total carbs: 4g; Net carbs: 3g; Fiber: 1g; Sugar: 1g; Sodium: 371mg **Macros:** Fat: 77%; Protein: 19%; Carbs: 4%

BROCCOLI AND CAULIFLOWER RICE CASSEROLE

EGG-FREE, GLUTEN-FREE, NUT-FREE
Serves 4 / Prep time: 5 minutes / Cook time: 10 minutes

Broccoli and rice is a recipe many parents turn to when introducing their children to broccoli. Rice is off the menu for anyone on a ketogenic diet, but cauliflower rice is a wonderful substitute. Also, broccoli rice is so tiny, your kids won't even know they are eating vegetables!

2 tablespoons grass-fed butter

1 garlic clove, minced

3 cups frozen cauliflower rice

1 cup frozen broccoli rice

½ teaspoon salt

¼ teaspoon freshly ground black pepper

1 cup grated sharp cheddar cheese

¼ cup cream cheese, at room temperature

1 to 2 tablespoons heavy (whipping) cream

1. In a medium skillet over medium-low heat, melt the butter.

2. Add the garlic and sauté for 2 minutes or until fragrant. Add the cauliflower rice, broccoli rice, salt, and pepper.

3. Cook the mixture for about 4 minutes, and then remove from the heat.

4. Stir in the cheddar cheese and cream cheese and thin the mixture to your desired consistency with the heavy cream.

5. Serve warm.

Prep tip: If you are unable to find broccoli rice in the frozen food aisle, here is how you can make it: Cut cooked and cooled broccoli into florets; then chop it finely or pulse it three or four times in a food processor or blender until the grains are the size of rice.

Per Serving **Calories:** 270; Fat: 22g; Protein: 11g; Total carbs: 7g; Net carbs: 4g; Fiber: 3g; Sugar: 2g; Sodium: 541mg **Macros:** Fat: 73%; Protein: 16%; Carbs: 11%

CAULIFLOWER FRIED RICE

DAIRY-FREE, GLUTEN-FREE, NUT-FREE
Serves 2 / Prep time: 2 minutes / Cook time: 10 minutes

This dish has so much flavor, you won't even know that it is a keto recipe. Fried rice is known as a common side dish for teriyaki chicken or shrimp, but it makes a wonderfully flavorful main meal. Frozen vegetables work perfectly here to make a simple and quick but tasty dish for busy weeknights.

1 tablespoon avocado oil

4 cups frozen cauliflower rice

1 cup frozen peas and carrots blend

½ tablespoon minced fresh ginger

2 tablespoons tamari sauce

2 tablespoons sesame oil

2 large eggs, beaten

2 scallions, finely chopped

1. In a medium skillet over medium-high heat, warm the avocado oil.

2. Add the cauliflower, peas and carrots, ginger, tamari sauce, and sesame oil. Cook until the vegetables are cooked thoroughly, 5 to 6 minutes.

3. Add the eggs and scramble them into the vegetables.

4. Divide the mixture between 2 serving dishes and top with the scallions before serving.

Per Serving **Calories:** 362; Fat: 26g; Protein: 14g; Total carbs: 18g; Net carbs: 10g; Fiber: 8g; Sugar: 8g; Sodium: 1160mg **Macros:** Fat: 65%; Protein: 15%; Carbs: 20%

MEXICAN ZUCCHINI HASH

EGG-FREE, GLUTEN-FREE, NUT-FREE

Serves 4 / Prep time: 5 minutes / Cook time: 10 minutes

This unique recipe has all the wonderful flavors of a Mexican dish and none of the carbs from rice, beans, or tortillas. Zucchini is considered low impact for a ketogenic diet due to its high water content, high fiber content, and low carb count. The cheese used in this recipe is queso blanco, *a white cheese that can be found at most grocery stores.*

2 tablespoons avocado oil

½ onion, diced

2 garlic cloves, minced

4 large zucchini, diced

½ teaspoon salt

¼ teaspoon freshly ground black pepper

1 teaspoon ground cumin

1 cup sliced button mushrooms

1 cup queso blanco cheese

2 avocados, diced

2 tablespoons chopped fresh cilantro

1. In a large skillet over medium-high heat, warm the avocado oil.

2. Add the onion, garlic, and zucchini, and season with the salt, pepper, and cumin. Stir to mix.

3. Add the mushrooms and sauté for 4 to 6 minutes, or until the vegetables are soft.

4. Remove from the heat and top with the queso blanco, diced avocado, and cilantro. Serve warm.

Leftovers tip: Store leftover hash in an airtight container in the refrigerator for up to 3 days.

Per Serving **Calories:** 401; Fat: 29g; Protein: 12g; Total carbs: 23g; Net carbs: 13g; Fiber: 10g; Sugar: 8g; Sodium: 361mg **Macros:** Fat: 65%; Protein: 13%; Carbs: 22%

EGGPLANT LASAGNA

GLUTEN-FREE, NUT-FREE

Serves 4 / Prep time: 10 minutes / Cook time: 1 hour 10 minutes

Lasagna is justifiably one of America's (and Italy's) favorite dishes. In order to still be able to enjoy it on a vegetarian ketogenic diet, the carb-heavy noodles are replaced by eggplant. The zucchini adds a unique flavor and keeps the carbs low. If you don't enjoy the taste of eggplant, you can use zucchini instead.

Nonstick cooking spray

1 large eggplant, cut into ⅛-inch-thick slices

Salt

1½ cups full-fat ricotta cheese

1 large egg

1 (28-ounce) can whole tomatoes, drained

1 cup grated Parmesan cheese

2 cups shredded mozzarella cheese

2 tablespoons dried parsley

1. Preheat the oven to 375°F. Grease an 8-by-8-inch baking dish with cooking spray.

2. Sprinkle the eggplant slices with salt. Allow them to sit for 15 minutes and then blot with a paper towel.

3. In a dry skillet over high heat, cook the eggplant slices for 3 minutes on each side. Remove and set aside.

4. In a medium bowl, combine the ricotta cheese and egg, and stir well. Set aside.

5. Crush a handful of tomatoes and place them in the bottom of the prepared baking dish. Layer a few slices of eggplant, a layer of cheese sauce, and another layer of crushed tomatoes. Repeat this layering until the dish is full.

6. Sprinkle the Parmesan and mozzarella cheeses on top, followed by the parsley.

7. Cover the dish with aluminum foil and bake for 40 minutes. Remove the foil and bake for an additional 10 minutes.

8. Remove the lasagna from the oven and let it sit for 5 minutes before cutting and serving.

Prep tip: This can easily be made into a freezer meal by using an aluminum pan. Once you've finished step 5, cover the pan with plastic wrap and foil and store in the freezer for up to 1 month. Allow the lasagna to thaw in the refrigerator overnight before cooking at 375°F for 55 minutes.

Per Serving (¼ of dish) **Calories:** 439; Fat: 27g; Protein: 31g; Total carbs: 18g; Net carbs: 11g; Fiber: 7g; Sugar: 10g; Sodium: 726mg **Macros:** Fat: 55%; Protein: 28%; Carbs: 17%

SPAGHETTI SQUASH BAKE

EGG-FREE, GLUTEN-FREE, NUT-FREE
Serves 4 / Prep time: 10 minutes / Cook time: 30 minutes

Next to cauliflower, spaghetti squash is one of the most popular options for low-carb "pasta." Spaghetti squash is loaded with vitamins, minerals, antioxidants, and fiber, making it perfect for a ketogenic diet. Here it is paired with a rich and creamy Alfredo sauce and plenty of garlic and black pepper, giving this dish tons of flavor.

Nonstick cooking spray

1 tablespoon grass-fed butter

5 garlic cloves, minced

½ cup water

1 teaspoon seasoned vegetable base

1 cup heavy (whipping) cream

4 cups cooked and shredded
  spaghetti squash

½ cup grated Parmesan cheese

½ cup shredded mozzarella cheese

2 tablespoons chopped fresh parsley

1 teaspoon freshly ground black pepper

1. Preheat the oven to 350°F. Spray an 8-by-8-inch glass casserole dish with cooking spray.

2. In a medium saucepan over medium-low heat, melt the butter. Add the garlic and cook until fragrant, 2 to 3 minutes.

3. Add the water, vegetable base, and cream. Cook until well combined, and then remove from the heat.

4. Place the squash in the bottom of the prepared dish. Pour the cream mixture on top, and then top with the Parmesan and mozzarella cheeses, parsley, and pepper.

5. Bake for 20 minutes and serve warm.

Prep tip: Here's how to prepare spaghetti squash: Preheat the oven to 400°F. Chop the tip and tail off the squash, cut it in half lengthwise, and scoop out and discard the seeds. Rub 1 tablespoon of olive oil over the flesh of each half. Sprinkle with salt and pepper. Place the squash cut-side down on a baking sheet lined with aluminum foil. Roast it for 35 to 50 minutes, or until the flesh is tender. When the squash is cool enough to handle, use a fork to gently scrape the flesh, releasing spaghetti-like strands. Place the "spaghetti" in an airtight container and store in the refrigerator.

Per Serving **Calories:** 371; Fat: 31g; Protein: 11g; Total carbs: 12g; Net carbs: 11g; Fiber: 1g; Sugar: 0g; Sodium: 461mg **Macros:** Fat: 75%; Protein: 12%; Carbs: 13%

CHEESY SPINACH BAKE

GLUTEN-FREE, NUT-FREE

Serves 4 / Prep time: 10 minutes / Cook time: 40 minutes

There is a reason that Popeye ate spinach like it was going out of style: Spinach is rich in carotenoids, a source of vitamin K, and high in vitamin C. Spinach is also one of the vegetables that has a neutral flavor once cooked and takes on the flavor of the food it is mixed with. This cheesy spinach bake is loaded with flavor, healthy fats, and, of course, spinach!

Nonstick cooking spray

2 tablespoons grass-fed butter

2 cups chopped onion

2 garlic cloves, minced

2 zucchinis, chopped into bite-size pieces

2 cups fresh spinach

3 eggs, beaten

¼ cup heavy (whipping) cream

½ teaspoon salt

¼ teaspoon freshly ground black pepper

1½ cups shredded mozzarella cheese

½ cup grated Parmesan cheese

1. Preheat the oven to 350°F. Coat a 9-inch glass pie plate with cooking spray.

2. In a skillet over medium-high heat, melt the butter. Add the onion and garlic and sauté for 2 minutes.

3. Add the zucchini and cook for another 4 minutes. Add the spinach and stir until wilted. Transfer the mixture to the prepared pie plate and spread it evenly with a spatula.

4. In a small bowl, mix together the eggs, cream, salt, and pepper. Pour the mixture over the vegetables.

5. Top with the mozzarella and Parmesan cheeses and bake for 30 to 35 minutes. Serve warm.

Per Serving **Calories:** 386; Fat: 30g; Protein: 21g; Total carbs: 8g; Net carbs: 6g; Fiber: 2g; Sugar: 3g; Sodium: 736mg **Macros:** Fat: 70%; Protein: 22%; Carbs: 8%

FAKEACHINI ALFREDO

EGG-FREE, NUT-FREE

Serves 1 / Prep time: 15 minutes / Cook time: 5 minutes

Even though pasta is totally off-limits on a ketogenic diet, using substitutes such as spaghetti squash can trick your taste buds into thinking you're actually eating pasta. This dish, with its rich and cheesy flavors, will quench those pasta cravings. Having cooked spaghetti squash on hand (see page 109) makes this dish a snap to prepare.

½ tablespoon extra-virgin olive oil

1 teaspoon minced garlic

¼ teaspoon salt

¼ teaspoon garlic powder

1 wedge Laughing Cow Swiss cheese, cubed

1 to 2 tablespoons heavy (whipping) cream

3 tablespoons grated Parmesan cheese

2 ounces seitan strips or cubes

⅓ cup cooked spaghetti squash

1 tablespoon chopped fresh parsley

1. In a small saucepan over medium-low heat, warm the olive oil. Add the garlic, salt, and garlic powder and stir for 1 to 2 minutes or until fragrant.

2. Add the cubed cheese and stir until melted. Thin the sauce to your desired consistency with the cream. Lower the heat and stir in the Parmesan cheese. Continue to stir until melted.

3. Add the seitan to the sauce.

4. Place the squash in a serving bowl, pour the sauce on top, and sprinkle with the parsley.

Per Serving **Calories:** 452; Fat: 24g; Protein: 52g; Total carbs: 7g; Net carbs: 4g; Fiber: 3g; Sugar: 1g; Sodium: 1887mg **Macros:** Fat: 48%; Protein: 46%; Carbs: 6%

CHEESY CAULIFLOWER MAC 'N' CHEESE

EGG-FREE, GLUTEN-FREE, NUT-FREE
Serves 6 / Prep time: 10 minutes / Cook time: 30 minutes

An all-American staple, macaroni and cheese is one of the most comforting foods around. Happily, being on a ketogenic diet doesn't mean you have to miss out on all that cheesy goodness. Cauliflower is a low-carb and tasty substitute for elbow macaroni. Use the cheeses as suggested, or try others for variety.

Nonstick cooking spray

1 cauliflower head, chopped into small florets

8 ounces heavy (whipping) cream

4 ounces shredded sharp cheddar cheese

4 ounces grated Parmesan cheese

2 ounces cream cheese

1 teaspoon salt

¼ teaspoon freshly ground black pepper

1. Preheat the oven to 375°F. Spray an 8-by-8-inch baking dish with cooking spray.

2. Place the cauliflower in a microwave-safe bowl and cook for 3 minutes on high. Drain any excess liquid.

3. In a small saucepan over medium heat, combine the heavy cream, cheddar cheese, Parmesan cheese, cream cheese, salt, and pepper. Stir until well combined, and then remove from the heat.

4. Pour the cheese sauce over the cauliflower and toss to coat. Transfer the mixture to the prepared baking dish and cook for 25 minutes.

Prep tip: If you wish to have the top nice and browned, cook the dish for 23 minutes and then place under low broil for the final 2 minutes.

Per Serving (½ cup) **Calories:** 324; Fat: 28g; Protein: 13g; Total carbs: 5g; Net carbs: 4g; Fiber: 1g; Sugar: 1g; Sodium: 737mg **Macros:** Fat: 78%; Protein: 16%; Carbs: 6%

MARGHERITA PIZZA

GLUTEN-FREE, NUT-FREE,
Serves 1 / Prep time: 10 minutes / Cook time: 5 minutes

This pizza recipe has a secret ingredient: psyllium husk powder, which is derived from a plant and is a great source of fiber. Psyllium is popular with many for its ability to help move things along in the digestive tract. Plus, it makes a delicious low-carb pizza crust.

1 tablespoon psyllium husk powder

¼ teaspoon salt

½ teaspoon dried oregano

2 large eggs

1 tablespoon avocado oil

3 tablespoons low-sugar marinara sauce

2 tablespoons grated Parmesan cheese

½ cup sliced mozzarella cheese

1 tablespoon chopped fresh basil

1. Line a baking sheet with aluminum foil. Turn the oven to low broil.

2. Combine the psyllium husk powder, salt, oregano, and eggs in a blender. Blend for 30 seconds. Set aside.

3. In a sauté pan or skillet, over high heat, warm the avocado oil. Pour the crust mixture into the pan, spreading it out into a circle.

4. Cook until the edges are browned, then flip the crust and cook for an additional minute.

5. Transfer the crust to the prepared baking sheet. Spread the marinara sauce over the top and cover with the Parmesan and mozzarella cheeses.

6. Broil until the cheese is melted and bubbling.

7. Top with the basil and enjoy.

Prep tip: If you prefer to prep your food ahead of time, the crusts can be made in bulk and stored in the refrigerator, wrapped in plastic wrap, for up to 3 days.

Per Serving **Calories:** 545; Fat: 41g; Protein: 32g; Total carbs: 12g; Net carbs: 4g; Fiber: 8g; Sugar: 2g; Sodium: 1252mg **Macros:** Fat: 68%; Protein: 23%; Carbs: 9%

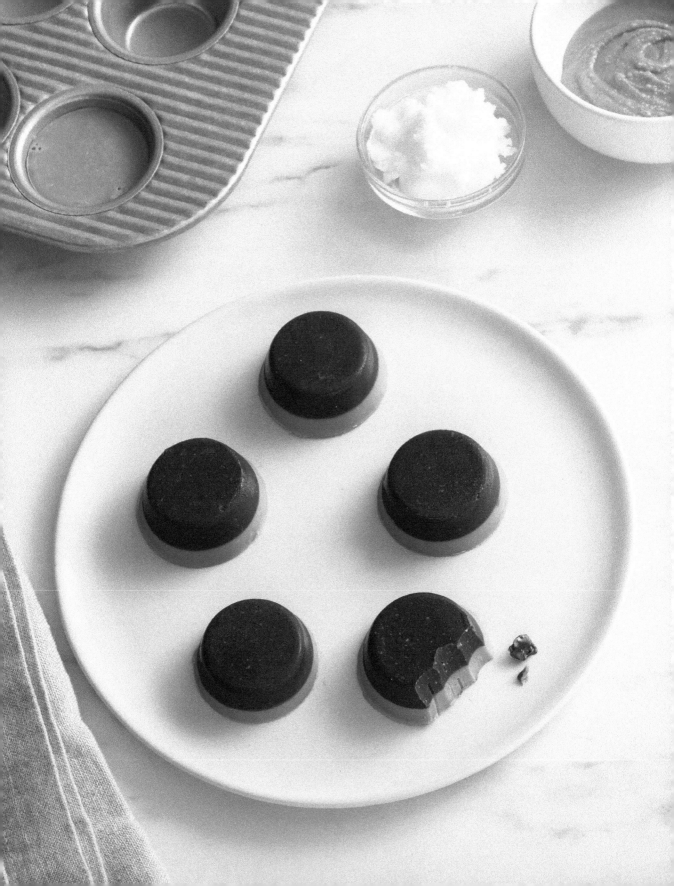

CHAPTER EIGHT

Desserts

Chocolate Sea Salt Almonds 116

Salted Caramel Cashew Brittle 117

Cookies and Cream Parfait 118

Pecan Pie Pudding 119

Chocolate Avocado Pudding 120

"Frosty" Chocolate Shake 121

French Vanilla Ice Cream with Hot Fudge 122

Cookie Dough 123

No-Bake Coconut Cookies 124

Lemon Bars 125

Peanut Butter Cookies 126

Fudge Brownies 127

Walnut Zucchini Bread 128

▶ Chocolate Peanut Butter Cups 129

Keto-Friendly Key Lime Pie 130

Mint Chocolate Fat Bombs 132

Keto Cheesecake 133

Strawberry Cheesecake Fat Bombs 135

CHOCOLATE SEA SALT ALMONDS

EGG-FREE, GLUTEN-FREE
Serves 8 / Prep time: 10 minutes, plus 30 minutes chill time

Chocolate, salt, and nuts. Simple and absolutely delicious. Sugar-free, low-carb melting chocolate can be found online and at specialty stores. I prefer Lily's dark chocolate brand, which is highly popular within the keto community.

4 ounces low-carb chocolate, chopped

1 tablespoon coconut oil

1 cup dry-roasted almonds

Sea salt

1. Line a rimmed baking sheet with parchment paper.

2. In a small saucepan over medium-low heat, melt the chocolate and coconut oil together while stirring constantly. Remove from the heat once melted and pour into a small bowl.

3. Add the almonds to the chocolate and give them a good stir.

4. Using a teaspoon, remove a cluster of almonds and place it on the prepared baking sheet. Immediately sprinkle with a bit of sea salt.

5. Repeat step 4 with the remaining nuts.

6. Place the baking sheet in the refrigerator for 30 minutes or until set.

7. Remove and store the clusters in small resealable plastic bags (or cover each cluster with plastic wrap) in the refrigerator until ready to eat.

Change it up: Any nuts can be used—macadamias, peanuts, pistachios, and cashews are all delicious.

Per Serving (1 cluster) **Calories:** 187; Fat: 15g; Protein: 6g; Total carbs: 7g; Net carbs: 3g; Fiber: 4g; Sugar: 1g; Sodium: 35mg **Macros:** Fat: 72%; Protein: 13%; Carbs: 15%

SALTED CARAMEL CASHEW BRITTLE

EGG-FREE, GLUTEN-FREE
Serves 6 / Prep time: 10 minutes / Cook time: 5 minutes, plus 1 hour chill time

Cashews are considered one of the most nutrient-dense nuts. They are high in essential minerals such as manganese, potassium, copper, iron, and selenium. These minerals can help lower blood pressure and harmful LDL cholesterol while increasing beneficial HDL cholesterol. Even though cashews are mostly used in savory recipes, they are wonderful with this keto-friendly caramel.

8 tablespoons grass-fed butter

4 tablespoons brown erythritol, granulated

4 ounces raw unsalted cashews

4 tablespoons natural cashew butter

Coarse sea salt

1. Line a rimmed baking sheet with parchment paper.

2. In a small saucepan over low heat, stir the butter until it melts.

3. Add the erythritol, cashews, and cashew butter. Mix until thoroughly combined and melted.

4. Pour the mixture onto the prepared baking sheet.

5. Sprinkle salt on top.

6. Place the baking sheet in the refrigerator to harden for about 1 hour.

7. Remove the brittle from the sheet and break into about 12 pieces.

8. Place each piece of brittle in a snack-size resealable plastic bag and store in the refrigerator or freezer for later use.

Per Serving (2 pieces) **Calories:** 321; Fat: 29g; Protein: 5g; Total carbs: 10g; Net carbs: 9g; Fiber: 1g; Sugar: 2g; Sodium: 197mg; Erythritol carbs: 8g **Macros:** Fat: 81%; Protein: 7%; Carbs: 12%

COOKIES AND CREAM PARFAIT

EGG-FREE, NUT-FREE
Serves 1 / Prep time: 5 minutes

This recipe is an example of how you can still eat normal foods, such as Oreos, on a ketogenic diet by keeping the portions in check. Here, you use just one side of an Oreo. You will still get the yummy chocolate crunch, but without using up too many carbs for the day. You know the saying "less is more"?

½ scoop low-carb vanilla protein powder

¾ cup plain full-fat Greek yogurt

1 Oreo cookie

4 tablespoons sugar-free chocolate syrup (I like Walden Farms)

1. In a small bowl, mix together the protein powder and Greek yogurt until smooth and creamy.

2. Remove one side of the Oreo cookie. Place it in a small resealable plastic bag and crush it with the back of a spoon. Set aside.

3. Pour the chocolate syrup over the yogurt mixture and sprinkle with the cookie crumbles.

Per Serving (1 parfait) **Calories:** 281; Fat: 13g; Protein: 19g; Total carbs: 22g; Net carbs: 19g; Fiber: 3g; Sugar: 16g; Sodium: 236mg **Macros:** Fat: 42%; Protein: 27%; Carbs: 31%

PECAN PIE PUDDING

EGG-FREE, GLUTEN-FREE
Serves 1 / Prep time: 5 minutes

This pudding is a favorite among low-carb dieters. It's quick and easy to prepare, and the flavor is reminiscent of a traditional holiday dish: pecan pie. The Greek yogurt provides a creamy base, and the pecans add flavor and crunch.

¾ cup plain full-fat Greek yogurt

½ scoop low-carb vanilla protein powder

4 tablespoons chopped pecans

2 tablespoons sugar-free syrup

1. In a small bowl, mix together the Greek yogurt and protein powder until smooth and creamy.

2. Top with the chopped pecans and syrup.

Ingredient tip: Walden Farms makes a tasty sugar-free syrup that should be easy to find.

Per Serving (1 parfait) **Calories:** 381; Fat: 21g; Protein: 32g; Total carbs: 16g; Net carbs: 9g; Fiber: 7g; Sugar: 6g; Sodium: 143mg **Macros:** Fat: 50%; Protein: 34%; Carbs: 16%

CHOCOLATE AVOCADO PUDDING

DAIRY-FREE, EGG-FREE, GLUTEN-FREE
Serves 1 / Prep time: 5 minutes

Avocados make the creamiest, most delicious puddings. They have a neutral flavor that can be easily blended with other flavors such as chocolate or cinnamon. This recipe will quickly become a weekly, if not daily, staple for your ketogenic diet.

1 avocado, halved

⅓ cup full-fat coconut milk

1 teaspoon vanilla extract

2 tablespoons unsweetened cocoa powder

5 or 6 drops liquid stevia

Combine all the ingredients in a high-powered blender or food processor and blend until smooth. Serve immediately.

Prep tip: For an ice cream–type treat, place the pudding in the freezer for 20 minutes, or until it reaches a soft-serve consistency.

Per Serving **Calories:** 555; Fat: 47g; Protein: 7g; Total carbs: 26g; Net carbs: 9g; Fiber: 17g; Sugar: 4g; Sodium: 29mg **Macros:** Fat: 76%; Protein: 5%; Carbs: 19%

"FROSTY" CHOCOLATE SHAKE

EGG-FREE, GLUTEN-FREE

Serves 2 / Prep time: 10 minutes, plus 30 minutes chill time

This recipe is a great way to make a classic all-American favorite treat into a keto dream. Make sure it has the consistency of whipped cream before placing it in the freezer, and it will turn out perfectly.

1 cup heavy (whipping) cream or
  coconut cream

2 tablespoons unsweetened cocoa powder

1 tablespoon almond butter

1 teaspoon vanilla extract

5 or 6 drops liquid stevia

1. In a medium bowl or using a stand mixer, beat the cream until fluffy, 3 to 4 minutes.

2. Add the cocoa powder, almond butter, vanilla, and stevia. Beat the mixture for an additional 2 to 3 minutes, or until the mixture has the consistency of whipped cream.

3. Place the bowl in the freezer for 25 to 30 minutes before serving.

Change it up: To make this dairy-free, simply replace the heavy cream with the same amount of coconut cream.

Per Serving **Calories:** 493; Fat: 49g; Protein: 5g; Total carbs: 8g; Net carbs: 5g; Fiber: 3g; Sugar: 1g; Sodium: 47mg **Macros:** Fat: 89%; Protein: 4%; Carbs: 7%

FRENCH VANILLA ICE CREAM WITH HOT FUDGE

EGG-FREE, GLUTEN-FREE
Serves 2 / Prep time: 10 minutes

This simple, five-ingredient recipe does take a bit of babysitting, but it will be more than worth it when you are enjoying a bowl of keto-friendly vanilla ice cream. Many homemade ice cream recipes require an ice cream machine to churn the ice cream base, but this one needs no special tools or ingredients.

1¼ cups heavy (whipping) cream, divided

¼ cup unsweetened almond milk

½ cup Swerve sweetener, divided

1½ teaspoons vanilla extract, divided

2 ounces unsweetened chocolate, chopped

1. Place a bread loaf pan in the freezer to chill for about 20 minutes.

2. In a medium bowl, combine ¾ cup of cream, the almond milk, ¼ cup of Swerve, and ½ teaspoon of vanilla.

3. Mix with a handheld electric mixer for 2 minutes, or until the sweetener has dissolved.

4. Pour the ice-cream mixture into the chilled loaf pan.

5. Place the pan in the freezer. Every half hour, remove the pan, scrape down the sides, and whisk the mixture for about 1 minute. It will get thicker and thicker each time you whisk it.

6. While the ice cream is in the freezer, combine the remaining ½ cup of cream, remaining ¼ cup of Swerve, and the chocolate in a double boiler over medium-low heat. Stir just until the chocolate melts, and then remove the mixture from the heat. Stir in the remaining 1 teaspoon of vanilla.

7. After 3½ to 4 hours, the ice cream will be thick enough to eat. Scrape down the sides for the last time and scoop out to serve. Pour the warm sauce over the ice cream.

Change it up: Varying the ice cream flavor is easy. For chocolate, add 2 tablespoons of cocoa powder, or for strawberry, add ¼ cup of finely chopped strawberries.

Per Serving (½ batch ice cream plus 2 tablespoons hot fudge) **Calories:** 719; Fat: 71g; Protein: 7g; Total carbs: 13g; Net carbs: 8g; Fiber: 5g; Sugar: 1g; Sodium: 109mg; Erythritol Carbs: 48g **Macros:** Fat: 89%; Protein: 4%; Carbs: 7%

COOKIE DOUGH

EGG-FREE, GLUTEN-FREE
Serves 18 to 20 / Prep time: 10 minutes, plus 15 minutes chill time

Cookie dough, often touted as the ultimate treat, is certainly not keto-friendly. But with a couple of tweaks, this version is now perfect for late-night cravings or midafternoon munchies. The butter is the base, so make sure to pick a good-quality, unsalted one.

8 tablespoons unsalted grass-fed butter, at
   room temperature

⅓ cup Swerve sweetener

½ teaspoon vanilla extract

¼ teaspoon salt

2 cups almond flour

½ cup dark chocolate chips

1. In the bowl of a stand mixer, combine the butter, Swerve, vanilla, and salt. Beat until the mixture is light and fluffy.

2. Add the almond flour and continue to mix on low until a dough forms.

3. Fold in the chocolate chips until just barely combined.

4. Place the dough in refrigerator for about 15 minutes to set. Line a baking sheet with parchment paper.

5. Using a 2-inch cookie scoop, scoop balls of dough onto the prepared baking sheet.

6. Store the cookie-dough balls in the refrigerator until ready to eat.

Per Serving (1 ball) **Calories:** 122; Fat: 10g; Protein: 2g; Total carbs: 6g; Net carbs: 5g; Fiber: 1g; Sugar: 4g; Sodium: 70mg: Erythritol Carbs: 4g **Macros:** Fat: 74%; Protein: 6%; Carbs: 20%

NO-BAKE COCONUT COOKIES

EGG-FREE, GLUTEN-FREE
Serves 12 / Prep time: 10 minutes / Cook time: 5 minutes,
plus 30 minutes chill time

These no-bake cookies are made with coconut flakes and sugar-free chocolate chips instead of the usual oats and sweetened chocolate, making this recipe a keto winner.

2 tablespoons grass-fed butter

⅔ cup crunchy natural peanut butter

1½ tablespoons unsweetened
  cocoa powder

5 or 6 drops liquid stevia

1 cup finely shredded unsweetened
  coconut flakes

1. Line a baking sheet with parchment paper.

2. In a medium saucepan over medium heat, melt the butter.

3. Add the peanut butter and cocoa powder, and stir well.

4. Remove from the heat and add the stevia. Stir in the coconut flakes and mix until all the ingredients are well combined.

5. Scoop the dough in small spoonfuls onto the prepared baking sheet.

6. Place the baking sheet in the refrigerator for 30 minutes to set.

7. Store the cookies in the refrigerator until ready to eat.

Change it up: To make the recipe dairy-free, replace the butter with an equal amount of coconut oil.

Per Serving (1 cookie) **Calories:** 153; Fat: 13g; Protein: 4g; Total carbs: 5g; Net carbs: 3g; Fiber: 2g; Sugar: 2g; Sodium: 75mg **Macros:** Fat: 76%; Protein: 11%; Carbs: 13%

LEMON BARS

DAIRY-FREE, GLUTEN-FREE
Serves 9 / Prep time: 15 minutes / Cook time: 25 minutes

Fruit is generally not suitable for a ketogenic diet, with the exception of limes, lemons, and a limited quantity of berries. Other fruits are too high in sugar and carbs to be part of your diet, but the good news is that delicious desserts are still perfectly possible. These lemon bars are simple to make but will help satisfy your craving for fruit.

Nonstick cooking spray

1⅛ cups almond flour

⅛ cup powdered erythritol sweetener, plus
 ⅔ cup, plus more for sprinkling

⅓ cup coconut oil, melted

2 large eggs

2 tablespoons plus 2 teaspoons freshly
 squeezed lemon juice

¼ teaspoon baking powder

½ tablespoon coconut flour

1. Preheat the oven to 350°F. Spray an 8-by-8-inch baking dish with cooking spray.

2. In a small bowl, combine the almond flour and ⅛ cup of erythritol. Add the melted coconut oil and blend until the mixture is crumbly.

3. Press the crust mixture into the bottom of the prepared baking dish. Bake for 10 minutes, or until the crust is slightly golden brown.

4. In a high-powered blender, combine the eggs, remaining ⅔ cup of erythritol, lemon juice, baking powder, and coconut flour, and blend for about 30 seconds.

5. Pour the filling into the crust and cook for an additional 10 to 12 minutes, or until the filling is set.

6. Remove from the oven and sprinkle with a dusting of powdered sweetener.

7. Allow to cool, then serve.

Per Serving (1 square) **Calories:** 128; Fat: 12g; Protein: 3g; Total carbs: 2g; Net carbs: 1g; Fiber: 1g; Sugar: 0g; Sodium: 19mg; Erythritol Carbs: 19g **Macros:** Fat: 84%; Protein: 9%; Carbs: 7%

PEANUT BUTTER COOKIES

DAIRY-FREE, GLUTEN-FREE
Serves 12 / Prep time: 10 minutes / Cook time: 10 minutes

Not all sweeteners are created equal. Some keto-friendly options are sweeter than others, so varying quantities are required to make a particular recipe work. The four most popular sweeteners are stevia, erythritol, monk fruit, and Swerve. If the recipe requires a powdered sweetener, any of these can be pulsed in a blender or food processor to create keto-approved powdered sugar.

Nonstick cooking spray
1 cup chunky natural peanut butter

¾ cup erythritol, granulated
1 egg, beaten

1. Preheat the oven to 350°F. Spray a baking sheet with cooking spray.

2. In a medium mixing bowl, combine the peanut butter and erythritol. Mix well.

3. Add the egg and stir until thoroughly combined.

4. Using a 2-inch cookie scoop, roll the dough into balls and set them on the prepared baking sheet.

5. Using the back of a fork, press a crisscross pattern onto the top of each cookie.

6. Bake for 9 to 10 minutes, then transfer to a wire rack to cool.

Change it up: Almond butter can be used in place of peanut butter for a different flavor.

Per Serving (1 cookie) **Calories:** 135; Fat: 11g; Protein: 5g; Total carbs: 4g; Net carbs: 3g; Fiber: 1g; Sugar: 1g; Sodium: 65mg; Erythritol Carbs: 12g **Macros:** Fat: 73%; Protein: 15%; Carbs: 12%

FUDGE BROWNIES

GLUTEN-FREE

Serves 12 / Prep time: 15 minutes / Cook time: 20 minutes

Conventional brownies are made with sugar and white flour, which are off-limits on keto, but there are many keto-friendly substitutes easily available that will help keep your carbs in check. These brownies are a perfect Sunday-night treat; try them with a dollop of peanut butter on top!

Nonstick cooking spray

12 tablespoons (1½ sticks) grass-fed butter

2 ounces dark chocolate squares (80 percent or higher), broken into chunks

¼ cup unsweetened cocoa powder

½ cup almond flour

⅔ cup Swerve sweetener

½ teaspoon baking powder

3 large eggs, beaten

1. Preheat the oven to 350°F. Grease an 8-by-8-inch baking dish with cooking spray.

2. In a small saucepan over low heat, melt the butter and dark chocolate while stirring. When melted, add the cocoa powder and stir until combined. Set aside.

3. In a small mixing bowl, combine the almond flour, Swerve, and baking powder. Stir well.

4. In a separate bowl, pour in the eggs and then slowly stir in the dark chocolate mixture. Mix together for about 1 minute to make sure everything is well combined.

5. Pour the flour mixture into the chocolate mixture and stir until a batter forms.

6. Spread the batter into the prepared baking dish and cook for 18 to 20 minutes, or until a toothpick inserted into the center comes out clean.

7. Remove from the oven and allow to cool before cutting into 12 squares.

Leftovers tip: Wrap each brownie in plastic wrap and store in the refrigerator until ready to eat.

Per Serving (1 brownie) **Calories:** 163; Fat: 15g; Protein: 3g; Total carbs: 4g; Net carbs: 3g; Fiber: 1g; Sugar: 2g; Sodium: 102mg; Erythritol Carbs: 11g **Macros:** Fat: 83%; Protein: 7%; Carbs: 10%

WALNUT ZUCCHINI BREAD

GLUTEN-FREE

Serves 9 / Prep time: 15 minutes / Cook time: 1 hour

In July and August, zucchini season is in full swing, and it's always fun to come up with new ways to eat it. Zucchini is a versatile vegetable that can be used in everything from noodles and stir-fries to muffins and cookies. This recipe is a staple when doing keto, especially when zucchini is abundant.

Nonstick cooking spray

2 cups almond flour

½ teaspoon ground cinnamon

1 teaspoon baking soda

2 large eggs

⅓ cup grass-fed butter, at room
temperature

½ cup erythritol, granulated

1½ cups grated and squeezed dry zucchini

⅓ cup sugar-free chocolate chips

1. Preheat the oven to 350°F. Grease a bread loaf pan with cooking spray.

2. In a medium bowl, sift together the almond flour, cinnamon, and baking soda. Set aside.

3. In the bowl of a stand mixer, beat together the eggs, butter, and erythritol until combined, 1 to 2 minutes. Stir in the zucchini.

4. Slowly add the flour mixture to the egg mixture. Blend until only just combined.

5. Stir in the chocolate chips.

6. Pour the batter into the prepared loaf pan and cook for 1 hour, or until a toothpick inserted in the middle comes out clean.

Per Serving (1 slice) **Calories:** 175; Fat: 15g; Protein: 5g; Total carbs: 5g; Net carbs: 3g; Fiber: 2g; Sugar: 1g; Sodium: 211mg; Erythritol Carbs: 16g **Macros:** Fat: 78%; Protein: 11%; Carbs: 11%

CHOCOLATE PEANUT BUTTER CUPS

DAIRY-FREE, EGG-FREE, GLUTEN-FREE
Serves 6 / Prep time: 20 minutes

One of the secrets to staying motivated on a diet is to re-create some of your tried-and-true favorites into healthier versions. This recipe for chocolate peanut butter cups will keep you far away from the candy aisle at the store.

For the chocolate layer

Nonstick cooking spray

2 tablespoons coconut oil, melted

4 tablespoons creamy natural peanut butter

2 tablespoons unsweetened cocoa powder

4 or 5 drops liquid stevia

For the peanut butter layer

2 tablespoons coconut oil, melted

4 tablespoons natural peanut butter

¼ teaspoon vanilla extract

4 or 5 drops liquid stevia

To make the chocolate layer

1. Spray the cups of a 12-cup mini muffin pan with cooking spray.

2. In a small bowl, whisk together all the ingredients until well combined.

3. Fill the bottom of each muffin cup with about 2 teaspoons of the mixture. Place in the freezer to set for about 8 minutes.

To make the peanut butter layer

While the chocolate layer is freezing, in a small bowl, combine all the ingredients for the peanut butter layer and mix well.

To assemble the cups

1. Remove the muffin tin from the freezer and top each chocolate layer with 2 teaspoons of peanut butter mixture.

2. Place the muffin tin back in the freezer and freeze for a further 8 minutes.

3. Use a butter knife to remove the cups from the tin and place them in a resealable plastic freezer bag. Store in the freezer.

Change it up: Peanut butter can be replaced with any other nut butter, such as almond, cashew, or macadamia.

Per Serving (3 cups) **Calories:** 224; Fat: 20g; Protein: 5g; Total carbs: 5g; Net carbs: 3g; Fiber: 2g; Sugar: 2g; Sodium: 5mg **Macros:** Fat: 82%; Protein: 9%; Carbs: 9%

KETO-FRIENDLY KEY LIME PIE

GLUTEN-FREE

Serves 6 / Prep time: 10 minutes / Cook time: 15 minutes, plus 4 hours chill time

Most traditional key lime pies are made with limes, egg yolks, and sweetened condensed milk. This keto version is a simplified, healthier version that takes less time to make and has fewer ingredients but still has the same great key lime flavor. Feel free to use some stevia drops to sweeten the crust or filling, if needed.

For the crust

Nonstick cooking spray

2 tablespoons coconut oil, melted

1 cup almond flour

1 tablespoon coconut flour

1 egg

⅛ teaspoon salt

For the filling

2 tablespoons coconut flour

2 (14-ounce) cans coconut cream

⅓ cup freshly squeezed lime juice

Zest of 2 limes

For the topping

2 cups heavy cream, whipped
  (see Prep tip)

2 teaspoons erythritol, for the
  whipped cream

1. Preheat the oven to 350°F. Spray a 9-inch pie plate with cooking spray.

2. In the bowl of a food processor or a high-speed blender, combine the coconut oil, almond flour, coconut flour, egg, and salt. Pulse until crumbly.

3. Pour the mixture into the prepared pie plate and use a fork to press the crust down evenly.

4. Bake for about 12 minutes, then set aside to cool for 10 minutes.

5. While the crust is cooling, in a medium bowl, use a hand mixer to mix together the coconut flour, coconut cream, lime juice, and lime zest for 1 to 2 minutes.

6. Pour the filling into the cooled crust and cover with plastic wrap.

7. Refrigerate for at least 4 hours to set.

8. Remove, slice, and top with the whipped cream.

Prep tip: To make a keto-friendly whipped cream, pour the heavy cream into a medium mixing bowl. Add the erythritol and use a hand mixer to whip the mixture slowly for about 2 minutes. Increase the mixer speed and mix the cream for an additional 3 to 5 minutes until soft peaks form. Store any unused cream in an airtight container in the refrigerator for up to 2 days.

Per Serving (1 slice) **Calories:** 814; Fat: 83g; Protein: 10g; Total carbs: 17g; Net carbs: 11g; Fiber: 6g; Sugar: 1g; Sodium: 127mg; Erythritol Carbs: 1g **Macros:** Fat: 87%; Protein: 4%; Carbs: 9%

MINT CHOCOLATE FAT BOMBS

DAIRY-FREE, EGG-FREE, GLUTEN-FREE
Serves 6 / Prep time: 10 minutes

Fat bombs come in all shapes, sizes, colors, and flavors. They are great to have on hand, not only as a treat but also to help you reach your daily fat macros. These minty treats are just sweet enough to satisfy sugar cravings and can be enjoyed after a meal or a snack.

⅔ cup coconut oil, melted

1 tablespoon erythritol, granulated

¼ teaspoon peppermint extract

2 tablespoons unsweetened cocoa powder

1. In a small mixing bowl, mix together the coconut oil, erythritol, and peppermint extract.

2. Use a silicone mold or an ice cube tray and fill six of the cups only halfway with the mixture. Note: You will have mixture left in the bowl.

3. Place the mold in the refrigerator for 5 minutes.

4. Add the cocoa powder to the remaining mixture and stir well.

5. Pour a cocoa layer on top of each peppermint layer and place the mold back in the refrigerator until set.

6. Use a butter knife to remove the bombs from the mold (they should just pop right out) and place them in a resealable freezer bag. Store in the refrigerator or freezer.

Per Serving (1 fat bomb) **Calories:** 229; Fat: 25g; Protein: 0g; Total carbs: 1g; Net carbs: 0g; Fiber: 1g; Sugar: 0g; Sodium: 0mg; Erythritol Carbs: 2g **Macros:** Fat: 98%; Protein: 0%; Carbs: 2%

KETO CHEESECAKE

GLUTEN-FREE

Serves 6 / Prep time: 30 minutes / Cook time: 1 hour, 5 minutes

Classic New York cheesecake is given a keto spin with a nut crust instead of a traditional graham-cracker crust. It has a wonderful keto-friendly strawberry topping that you can also use on keto ice cream or pancakes.

For the crust

2 cups almond flour

⅓ cup butter, melted

2 tablespoons granulated erythritol

1 teaspoon vanilla extract

For the filling

32 ounces cream cheese, at room
  temperature

1 cup powdered erythritol

3 large eggs

1 tablespoon freshly squeezed lemon juice

1 teaspoon vanilla extract

For the topping

1 cup diced strawberries

½ tablespoon freshly squeezed lemon juice

¼ cup granulated erythritol

To make the crust

1. Preheat the oven to 350°F. Spray a 9-inch springform pan with cooking spray.

2. In a medium bowl, stir together the almond flour, butter, erythritol, and vanilla until a crumbly dough forms.

3. Press the crust into the bottom of the prepared pan and bake for around 9 minutes. Remove and allow to cool.

To make the filling

1. In a separate bowl, use a handheld electric mixer to mix together the cream cheese and powdered erythritol until blended.

2. Add the eggs and continue to beat until well combined.

3. Add the lemon juice and vanilla and beat for another minute.

4. Pour the filling into the cooled pie crust. Bake for 45 minutes, then set on a rack to cool.

CONTINUED

To make the topping

1. While the cheesecake is cooling, in a small saucepan over medium-low heat, stir together the topping ingredients and simmer, stirring occasionally, for 15 to 20 minutes.

2. Remove from the heat and allow to cool to room temperature. Then place the topping in a blender or food processor and pulse 5 to 7 times.

3. Transfer the sauce to a small bowl and serve alongside the cheesecake.

Per Serving (1 slice with 2 tablespoons strawberry sauce) **Calories:** 782; Fat: 74g; Protein: 19g; Total carbs: 10g; Net carbs: 7g; Fiber: 3g; Sugar: 2g; Sodium: 563mg; Erythritol Carbs: 44g **Macros:** Fat: 85%; Protein: 10%; Carbs: 5%

STRAWBERRY CHEESECAKE FAT BOMBS

EGG-FREE, GLUTEN-FREE, NUT-FREE
Serves 12 / Prep time: 10 minutes, plus 4 hours freeze time /
Cook time: 12 minutes

These decadent desserts take only a few minutes to make and can be varied according to whatever berries you have on hand. For best results, the berries need to be cooked ahead of time to release excess moisture. This will allow your fat bombs to mold correctly.

Nonstick cooking spray

⅓ cup frozen strawberries

4½ tablespoons cream cheese

4½ tablespoons grass-fed butter

2 tablespoons powdered erythritol

½ teaspoon vanilla extract

1. Spray the cups of a 12-cup mini muffin tin with cooking spray.

2. In a small saucepan over low heat, bring the strawberries to a simmer and cook for 10 minutes while stirring, until all the excess liquid has evaporated, leaving just the strawberries. Set aside.

3. In the bowl of a stand mixer, combine the cream cheese, butter, erythritol, and vanilla, and mix on low for 3 to 4 minutes or until fluffy.

4. Pour in the strawberries and mix for another 1 to 2 minutes.

5. Using a 2-inch cookie scoop, scoop the mixture into the mini muffin cups.

6. Place the muffin tin in the freezer to set for 4 hours.

7. Use a butter knife to remove the bombs from the tin (they should just pop right out) and place the bombs in a resealable freezer bag. Store in the freezer.

Leftovers tip: Before serving, allow the fat bomb to "defrost" for 5 to 10 minutes.

Per Serving (1 fat bomb) **Calories:** 58; Fat: 6g; Protein: 0g; Total carbs: 1g; Net carbs: 1g; Fiber: 0g; Sugar: 0g; Sodium: 42mg; Erythritol Carbs: 2g **Macros:** Fat: 93%; Protein: 0%; Carbs: 7%

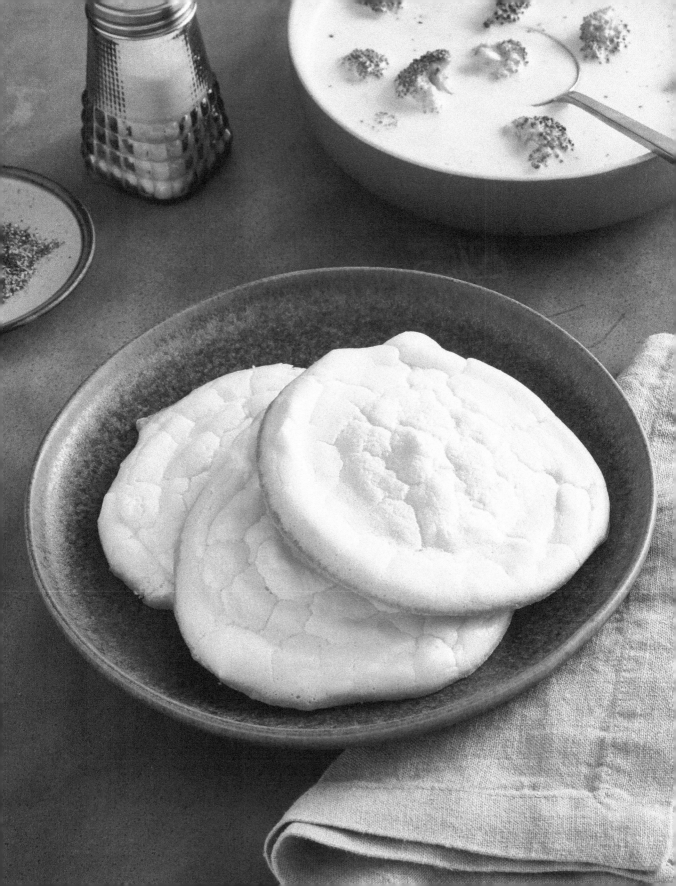

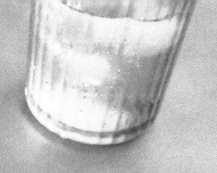

CHAPTER NINE

Staples, Sauces, and Dressings

Avocado Pesto Zoodles *138*

Cauliflower Rice *139*

Avocado Lime Dressing *140*

Quick and Easy Ranch Dip *141*

Coconut Iced Coffee *142*

Easy Keto Bread *143*

▶ Cloud Bread *144*

Fathead Crackers *145*

Queso Blanco Dip *146*

Classic Buttermilk Syrup *147*

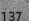

AVOCADO PESTO ZOODLES

EGG-FREE, GLUTEN-FREE
Serves 2 / Prep time: 10 minutes / Cook time: 10 minutes

Zucchini is one of the must-have vegetables when eating a ketogenic diet. It is versatile, low carb, and easily found year-round. Zoodles are made by spiralizing zucchini using a spiralizer or even just a vegetable peeler. The one thing to watch out for is overcooking, which leads to soggy zoodles. See the tip for how to make a tender, tasty zoodle without the extra water.

2 avocados, halved

1 tablespoon pine nuts

½ cup fresh basil

2 teaspoons olive oil

4 medium zucchini, spiralized

1 tablespoon minced garlic

4 tablespoons shredded Parmesan cheese

½ teaspoon salt

½ teaspoon freshly ground black pepper

1. In the bowl of a food processor, combine the avocados, pine nuts, and basil. Pulse until a paste forms, using a few tablespoons of water to thin the consistency if necessary.

2. Heat a medium skillet over medium-high heat and pour in the olive oil. Add the zoodles and garlic and sauté for 5 to 7 minutes.

3. Add the avocado pesto to the skillet and stir until well combined.

4. Cook for an additional 1 to 2 minutes and top with the Parmesan cheese, salt, and pepper.

Prep tip: Perfect zoodles are easy to make and can be used in any keto recipe in place of starchy pasta. Here is how to make them. Spiralize 1 zucchini and place in a colander. Sprinkle with ½ teaspoon of salt and let sit for 10 minutes. Pat dry with paper towels. Heat a small skillet over medium-high heat. Pour in 1 tablespoon of olive oil and add the zoodles. Sauté for 5 to 7 minutes. Remove the zoodles immediately and season.

Per Serving **Calories:** 404; Fat: 31g; Protein: 14g; Total carbs: 27g; Net carbs: 13g; Fiber: 14g; Sugar: 7g; Sodium: 766mg **Macros:** Fat: 65%; Protein: 11%; Carbs: 24%

CAULIFLOWER RICE

EGG-FREE, GLUTEN-FREE, NUT-FREE
Serves 2 / Prep time: 15 minutes / Cook time: 10 minutes

Cauliflower is an all-star vegetable in a keto diet. From pizza to breadsticks to pitas, cauliflower can be turned into just about any low-carb alternative dish. Frozen cauliflower rice is easily found at most grocery stores, but making it from scratch is simple.

½ head cauliflower

1 tablespoon grass-fed butter

½ teaspoon salt

⅛ teaspoon freshly ground black pepper

1. Wash the cauliflower under cold water. Pat dry with paper towels.

2. Chop the cauliflower into 1-inch pieces and put in a food processor. Pulse until the size of small rice.

3. Place a small griddle over medium-high heat. Melt the butter and add the cauliflower. Season with the salt and pepper and cook for 7 to 8 minutes, or until the cauliflower is tender.

Change it up: To make cheesy cauliflower rice, follow the recipe as written; then turn heat to low and stir in 2 tablespoons of cream cheese, 2 tablespoons of milk, and 1 cup of grated cheddar cheese. Stir until everything is melted and warm.

Per Serving **Calories:** 74; Fat: 6g; Protein: 1g; Total carbs: 4g; Net carbs: 2g; Fiber: 2g; Sugar: 2g; Sodium: 642mg **Macros:** Fat: 73%; Protein: 5%; Carbs: 22%

AVOCADO LIME DRESSING

DAIRY-FREE, EGG-FREE, GLUTEN-FREE, NUT-FREE
Serves 6 / Prep time: 5 minutes

Everyone needs a staple dressing that tastes good on just about everything. This avocado lime dressing fits the bill and is super easy to make in just a few minutes. It's wonderful on anything from fajita veggies to scrambled eggs or drizzled over your favorite salad.

1 avocado, halved

Leaves of 1 bunch fresh cilantro

¼ cup avocado oil

2 tablespoons water

2 tablespoons freshly squeezed lime juice

1 garlic clove, peeled

1 teaspoon garlic salt

Combine all the ingredients in a high-powered blender or a food processor and pulse until thoroughly combined, 2 to 3 minutes. Transfer to a small mason jar and store in the refrigerator until ready to use.

Leftovers tip: This dressing can be stored, covered, for up to 5 days. Before serving, shake well.

Per Serving (2 tablespoons) **Calories:** 146; Fat: 14g; Protein: 1g; Total carbs: 4g; Net carbs: 2g; Fiber: 2g; Sugar: 0g; Sodium: 51mg **Macros:** Fat: 86%; Protein: 3%; Carbs: 11%

QUICK AND EASY RANCH DIP

EGG-FREE, GLUTEN-FREE, NUT-FREE
Serves 12 / Prep time: 10 minutes, plus 4 hours chill time

A classic buttermilk ranch should be part of any ketogenic diet. Use healthy fats to create a flavorful dressing to add to just about any vegetarian keto dish. Unlike most store-bought ranch seasonings and dressings, this recipe contains no MSG and can be made from pantry spices and buttermilk.

1 cup heavy (whipping) cream

1 tablespoon white distilled vinegar

¾ cup plain full-fat Greek yogurt

1 teaspoon freshly squeezed lemon juice

2 teaspoons dried parsley

1 teaspoon dried dill

1 teaspoon dried chives

½ teaspoon garlic powder

½ teaspoon onion powder

½ teaspoon salt

¼ teaspoon freshly ground black pepper

1. In a quart-size canning jar, combine the heavy cream and vinegar. Set aside for 5 minutes.

2. Add the Greek yogurt and lemon juice and stir (or shake the jar) well.

3. Add the parsley, dill, chives, garlic powder, onion powder, salt, and pepper, and stir until thoroughly mixed.

4. Put the lid on the jar and place in the refrigerator for 4 hours or overnight for the flavors to combine.

Per Serving (2 tablespoons) **Calories:** 79; Fat: 7g; Protein: 2g; Total carbs: 2g; Net carbs: 2g; Fiber: 0g; Sugar: 2g; Sodium: 109mg **Macros:** Fat: 80%; Protein: 10%; Carbs: 10%

COCONUT ICED COFFEE

EGG-FREE, GLUTEN-FREE, NUT-FREE
Serves 1 / Prep time: 5 minutes

Caffeine is not an essential part of the ketogenic diet, but it can be very helpful to use in the first few weeks of ketosis. When switching from glucose to ketones for your body's energy source, you can feel a bit fatigued or low-energy. This recipe is a great addition as a midafternoon energy boost to get you through the rest of the day.

Ice cubes

8 ounces brewed black coffee, chilled

5 drops monk fruit extract

1 teaspoon vanilla extract

1 teaspoon coconut extract

1 tablespoon MCT oil or powder

¼ cup heavy cream or coconut milk

1. Fill a large glass ¾ full of ice.

2. Pour the coffee over ice. Add the monk fruit, vanilla, and coconut extracts, and MCT oil and stir until combined.

3. Pour the heavy cream on top and allow to settle.

4. Serve cold.

Change it up: For a blended coffee drink, add ½ teaspoon ground cinnamon instead of the coconut extract and blend all the ingredients in a high-powered blender for 1 minute.

Per Serving **Calories:** 335; Fat: 36g; Protein: 1g; Total carbs: 2g; Net carbs: 2g; Fiber: 0g; Sugar: 0g; Sodium: 23mg **Macros:** Fat: 96%; Protein: 1%; Carbs: 3%

EASY KETO BREAD

DAIRY-FREE, GLUTEN-FREE
Makes 1 loaf / Prep time: 15 minutes / Cook time: 1 hour, 15 minutes

Yes, you can have bread on keto! This bread isn't made with white flour and sugar, but rather with egg whites as well as almond and coconut flours. Follow the recipe carefully, and after slicing off what you need, wrap the left-over loaf in plastic and store in the refrigerator.

Nonstick cooking spray

1 cup blanched almond flour

¼ cup coconut flour

2 teaspoons baking powder

¼ teaspoon salt

⅓ cup coconut oil, melted

12 egg whites

1. Preheat the oven to 350°F. Spray a loaf pan with cooking spray, making sure to cover the interior corners and sides completely.

2. In the bowl of a food processor, combine the almond flour, coconut flour, baking powder, and salt. Pulse until well combined.

3. Add the coconut oil and pulse again until a crumble forms. Set aside.

4. In a large bowl, use a handheld electric mixer to beat the egg whites until stiff peaks form, about 10 minutes. (You can add ¼ teaspoon of cream of tartar to help the egg whites whip up faster.)

5. Add half the whipped egg whites to the food processor. Pulse a few times. Don't overbeat or you will deflate the egg whites.

6. Bit by bit, add the flour mixture to the remaining egg whites in the large bowl. Fold the flour into the egg whites very gently until well combined.

7. Spread the batter in the prepared bread pan.

8. Bake for 40 minutes, or until the top of the bread is lightly browned.

9. Place a layer of aluminum foil over the top of the bread (to avoid overbrowning) and cook for an additional 35 minutes.

10. Transfer the bread to a wire rack. When cooled, slice evenly.

Ingredient tip: The temperature of the eggs matters. The colder they are, the better the results.

Per Serving (1 slice) **Calories:** 121; Fat: 9g; Protein: 5g; Total carbs: 5g; Net carbs: 2g; Fiber: 3g; Sugar: 0g; Sodium: 86mg **Macros:** Fat: 68%; Protein: 16%; Carbs: 16%

CLOUD BREAD

GLUTEN-FREE, NUT-FREE
Serves 6 / Prep time: 15 minutes / Cook time: 35 minutes

Keto cloud bread is unique because it mimics bread but has zero carbs. This useful bread is made with eggs and cream cheese whipped into stiff peaks and then baked. It can be used for pizza crusts or sandwich bread or dipped into a keto-approved soup.

Nonstick cooking spray

3 eggs, separated, at room temperature

3 ounces cream cheese, at room temperature

⅛ teaspoon salt

1. Preheat the oven to 300°F. Spray a baking sheet with cooking spray.

2. In a large mixing bowl, use a handheld electric mixer to beat the egg whites into stiff peaks. Set aside.

3. In a separate large bowl, combine the egg yolks, cream cheese, and salt, and mix until creamy.

4. Slowly pour the egg white mixture into the egg yolk mixture, and use a spatula to carefully fold it in. Be careful not to overmix.

5. Use the batter to make 6 separate circles on the prepared baking sheet. These will be your clouds.

6. Bake for 30 to 35 minutes or until golden brown.

7. Remove from the oven and allow to cool for 10 minutes before serving.

Per Serving (1 cloud) **Calories:** 82; Fat: 7g; Protein: 4g; Total carbs: 1g; Net carbs: 1g; Fiber: 0g; Sugar: 0g; Sodium: 123mg **Macros:** Fat: 76%; Protein: 19%; Carbs: 5%

FATHEAD CRACKERS

GLUTEN-FREE

Serves 4 / Prep time: 15 minutes / Cook time: 10 minutes

Fathead crackers are a keto-approved snack that can be used with many different meals. Enjoy these crackers with veggies on the side or a spread of cream cheese on the top. They are great with keto dips.

Nonstick cooking spray

1½ cups grated mozzarella cheese

⅔ cup almond flour

2 tablespoons cream cheese

1 egg

½ teaspoon salt

1. Preheat the oven to 425°F. Spray a baking sheet with cooking spray.

2. In a microwave-safe bowl, combine the mozzarella, almond flour, and cream cheese.

3. Microwave on high for 1 minute. Remove carefully and stir, then cook for an additional 30 seconds.

4. Remove the bowl and add the egg and salt. Stir quickly until a ball of dough forms.

5. Roll out the dough to ¼-inch thick. Olive oil can be used to avoid sticking.

6. Cut the dough into 1-inch squares. Use a spatula to carefully transfer the crackers to the prepared baking sheet.

7. Cook for 5 minutes. Flip and cook for another 5 minutes.

8. Transfer the crackers to a wire rack to cool.

Leftovers tip: These crackers can be stored in an airtight container for up to 3 days in the pantry.

Per Serving (6 crackers) **Calories:** 225; Fat: 18g; Protein: 13g; Total carbs: 3g; Net carbs: 2g; Fiber: 1g; Sugar: 1g; Sodium: 591mg **Macros:** Fat: 72%; Protein: 23%; Carbs: 5%

QUESO BLANCO DIP

EGG-FREE, GLUTEN-FREE, NUT-FREE
Serves 8 / Prep time: 5 minutes / Cook time: 10 minutes

One of the wonderful things about the keto diet is that delicious dips such as this queso blanco dip are allowed. The dip is low carb and high fat and lends itself for use with many keto dishes. Skip the chips, though, and pass the celery for happy dipping, or try the Fathead Crackers on page 145.

½ cup heavy (whipping) cream

3 ounces cream cheese

1 cup shredded Monterey Jack cheese

1 cup shredded queso blanco or other
   sharp white cheddar cheese

1 (4.5-ounce) can diced green chiles, drained

½ teaspoon freshly ground black pepper

½ teaspoon ground cumin

1. In a small saucepan over medium heat, melt together the heavy cream and cream cheese, whisking until totally melted.

2. Stir in the Monterey Jack cheese and queso blanco and the green chiles.

3. Remove from the heat and add the pepper and cumin.

4. Stir well and serve.

Per Serving (2 tablespoons) **Calories:** 202; Fat: 18g; Protein: 8g; Total carbs: 2g; Net carbs: 2g; Fiber: 0g; Sugar: 1g; Sodium: 265mg **Macros:** Fat: 80%; Protein: 16%; Carbs: 4%

CLASSIC BUTTERMILK SYRUP

EGG-FREE, GLUTEN-FREE, NUT-FREE
Serves 12 / Prep time: 5 minutes / Cook time: 10 minutes

Buttermilk syrup is often thought of as a major treat, or cheat, when on a diet. Most syrups are laden with sugar and are high in carbohydrates, which makes them unsuitable for a ketogenic diet. But with this recipe, you can have syrup on your Almond Butter Pancakes (page 45) or Chocolate Coconut "Oatmeal" (page 48). Made with heavy cream and keto-approved sweeteners, this recipe will sweeten your life.

¾ cup grass-fed butter

½ cup heavy (whipping) cream

¾ teaspoon white distilled vinegar

¼ cup water

1 cup powdered monk fruit

⅛ teaspoon salt

1 teaspoon baking soda

1 teaspoon vanilla extract

1. In a large saucepan over medium heat, melt the butter.

2. In a small bowl, mix together the heavy cream and vinegar. Allow to sit for 5 minutes.

3. Add the water and monk fruit to the butter, whisking until all the sweetener has dissolved.

4. Add the cream mixture and salt to the pan, continuing to whisk while bringing the mixture to a gentle boil.

5. Remove the pan from the heat and stir in the baking soda and vanilla. Keep an eye on it because it will foam up. Whisk until all the foam is gone.

6. Serve warm.

Change it up: Add ½ teaspoon of coconut extract to the syrup to add a more tropical flavor.

Per Serving (2 tablespoons) **Calories:** 137; Fat: 15g; Protein: 0g; Total carbs: 0g; Net carbs: 0g; Fiber: 0g; Sugar: 0g; Sodium: 133mg; Erythritol carbs: 16g **Macros:** Fat: 98%; Protein: 2%; Carbs: 0%

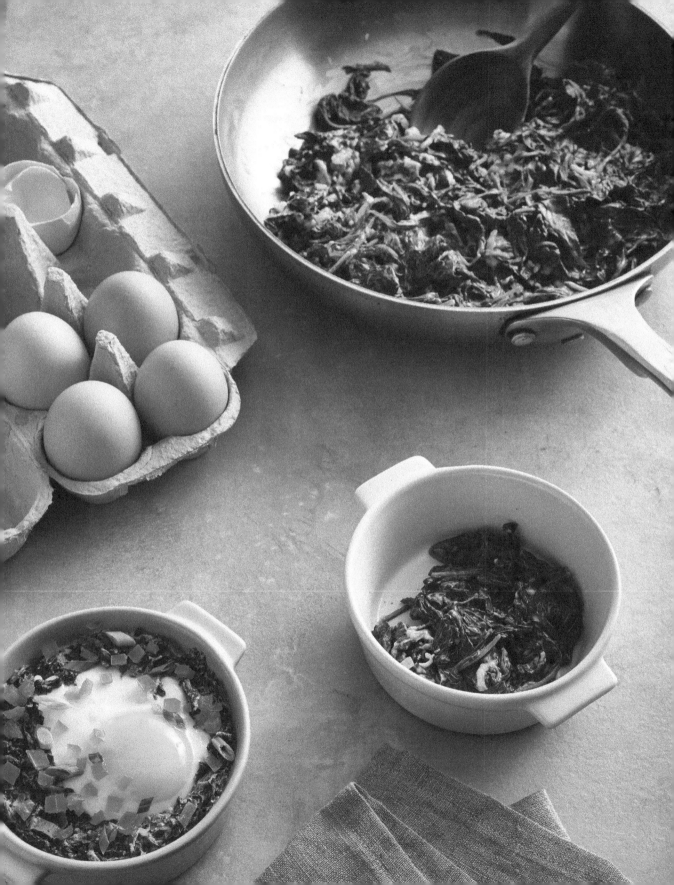

MEASUREMENT CONVERSIONS

Volume Equivalents (Liquid)

US Standard	US Standard (ounces)	Metric (approximate)
2 tablespoons	1 fl. oz.	30 mL
¼ cup	2 fl. oz.	60 mL
½ cup	4 fl. oz.	120 mL
1 cup	8 fl. oz.	240 mL
1½ cups	12 fl. oz.	355 mL
2 cups or 1 pint	16 fl. oz.	475 mL
4 cups or 1 quart	32 fl. oz.	1 L
1 gallon	128 fl. oz.	4 L

Oven Temperatures

Fahrenheit (F)	Celsius (C) (approximate)
250°F	120°C
300°F	150°C
325°F	165°C
350°F	180°C
375°F	190°C
400°F	200°C
425°F	220°C
450°F	230°C

Volume Equivalents (Dry)

US Standard	Metric (approximate)
⅛ teaspoon	0.5 mL
¼ teaspoon	1 mL
½ teaspoon	2 mL
¾ teaspoon	4 mL
1 teaspoon	5 mL
1 tablespoon	15 mL
¼ cup	59 mL
⅓ cup	79 mL
½ cup	118 mL
⅔ cup	156 mL
¾ cup	177 mL
1 cup	235 mL
2 cups or 1 pint	475 mL
3 cups	700 mL
4 cups or 1 quart	1 L

Weight Equivalents

US Standard	Metric (approximate)
½ ounce	15 g
1 ounce	30 g
2 ounces	60 g
4 ounces	115 g
8 ounces	225 g
12 ounces	340 g
16 ounces or 1 pound	455 g

RESOURCES

Blood Ketone Meter

FORA 6

This blood ketone meter will help accurately read your ketone levels each day with just a small prick of your finger.

Websites

CalorieKing: calorieking.com/us/en/

This comprehensive database can help you keep track of your macronutrient numbers.

Carb Manager: carbmanager.com

This keto tool has an ingredient database, recipes, meal plans, and shopping lists.

MyFitnessPal: myfitnesspal.com

The most widely used app for macronutrient tracking, MyFitnessPal lets you enter in your macronutrient goals and log the food you eat so you can know exactly what you can eat for the rest of the day.

INDEX

A

Alcohol, 9
Almond Butter Pancakes, 45
Artichokes
  Italian Vegetable
    Egg Bake, 42
Asparagus and Avocado
  Salad, 60
Avocados
  Avocado and Asparagus
    Salad, 60
  Avocado Egg Salad, 53
  Avocado Lime Dressing, 140
  Avocado Pesto Panini, 64
  Avocado Pesto Zoodles, 138
  Broccoli Stir-Fry, 98
  Caprese Stuffed Avocados, 82
  Chocolate Avocado
    Pudding, 120
  Flaxseed Chips and
    Guacamole, 80
  Green Goddess
    Buddha Bowl, 96
  Hemp Cobb Salad, 58
  Kale Refresher Smoothie, 32
  Loaded Bell Pepper
    Sandwich, 65
  Mexican Egg Casserole, 40–41
  Mexican Zucchini Hash, 107
  Portobello Mushroom
    Burger with Avocado, 70
  Roasted Cauliflower
    Lettuce Cups, 62
  Spinach Avocado Salad, 55
  Taco Lettuce Cups, 63

B

Bacon, vegan
  Eggs Benedict with Five-
    Minute Hollandaise, 43
  Hemp Cobb Salad, 58
Baked Olives, 86

Bell peppers
  Creamy Stuffed
    Peppers, 101
  Italian Vegetable
    Egg Bake, 42
  Loaded Bell Pepper
    Sandwich, 65
  Mediterranean Cucumber
    Bites, 76
  Mexican Egg Casserole, 40–41
  Taco Lettuce Cups, 63
Berries
  Keto Cheesecake, 133–134
  Strawberry Cheesecake
    Fat Bombs, 135
Beverages. *See also* Smoothies
  Coconut Iced Coffee, 142
  Fat Chai, 35
  Fat Coffee, 34
  Fat Hot Chocolate, 34–35
  Matcha Coffee, 36
Breads and crackers.
    See also Muffins
  Cheesy Cauliflower
    Breadsticks, 83–84
  Cheesy Crackers, 81
  Cloud Bread, 144
  Easy Keto Bread, 143
  Fathead Crackers, 145
  Flaxseed Chips and
    Guacamole, 80
  Walnut Zucchini Bread, 128
Broccoli
  Broccoli and Cauliflower
    Rice Casserole, 105
  Broccoli Quiche, 44
  Broccoli Stir-Fry, 98
  Slow Cooker Broccoli
    Cheese Soup, 67
Broccolini
  Green Goddess
    Buddha Bowl, 96

C

Cabbage
  Classic Creamy Coleslaw, 54
  Thai Noodle Salad, 61
Caprese Stuffed Avocados, 82
Carbohydrates, 3–4
Carrots
  Cauliflower Fried Rice, 106
  Green Goddess
    Buddha Bowl, 96
  Spinach Avocado Salad, 55
Cauliflower
  Broccoli and Cauliflower
    Rice Casserole, 105
  Broccoli Stir-Fry, 98
  Cauliflower Fried Rice, 106
  Cauliflower Rice, 139
  Cheesy Cauliflower
    Breadsticks, 83–84
  Cheesy Cauliflower Mac
    'n' Cheese, 112
  Creamed Cauliflower
    Soup, 69
  Green Goddess
    Buddha Bowl, 96
  Kale and Cashew Stir-Fry, 99
  Roasted Cauliflower
    Hummus, 77
  Roasted Cauliflower
    Lettuce Cups, 62
  Tofu Green Bean
    Casserole, 100
  Vegan Coconut Curry, 103
"Cheat days," 26–27
Cheese. *See also* Cottage
    cheese; Cream cheese;
    Ricotta cheese
  Avocado and Asparagus
    Salad, 60
  Avocado Pesto Panini, 64
  Avocado Pesto Zoodles, 138
  Baked Olives, 86

Cheese (*continued*)
  Broccoli and Cauliflower
    Rice Casserole, 105
  Broccoli Quiche, 44
  Caprese Stuffed
    Avocados, 82
  Cheesy Cauliflower
    Breadsticks, 83–84
  Cheesy Cauliflower Mac
    'n' Cheese, 112
  Cheesy Crackers, 81
  Cheesy Dill Fat Bombs, 92
  Cheesy Spinach Bake, 110
  Chiles Rellenos, 104
  Classic Club Salad, 57
  Creamed Cauliflower
    Soup, 69
  Creamed Spinach
    with Eggs, 39
  Creamy Spinach Dip, 78
  Creamy Stuffed Peppers, 101
  Eggplant Lasagna, 108
  "Everything But the Bagel"
    Fat Bombs, 91
  Fakeachini Alfredo, 111
  Fathead Crackers, 145
  Hemp Cobb Salad, 58
  Herbed Mozzarella Sticks, 85
  Instant Pot French
    Onion Soup, 68
  Loaded Bell Pepper
    Sandwich, 65
  Margherita Pizza, 113
  Mediterranean Salad, 59
  Mexican Egg
    Casserole, 40–41
  Mexican Zucchini Hash, 107
  Parmesan Zucchini
    Chips, 79
  Queso Blanco Dip, 146
  Roasted Garlic
    Mushrooms, 75
  Slow Cooker Broccoli
    Cheese Soup, 67
  Spaghetti Squash Bake, 109

Taco Lettuce Cups, 63
Three-Cheese Stuffed
  Mushrooms, 88
Tofu Green Bean
  Casserole, 100
Ultimate Grilled Cheese, 66
Zucchini Fritters, 87
Zucchini Sage Pasta, 97
Cheesy Cauliflower
  Breadsticks, 83–84
Cheesy Cauliflower Mac
  'n' Cheese, 112
Cheesy Crackers, 81
Cheesy Dill Fat Bombs, 92
Cheesy Spinach Bake, 110
Chiles Rellenos, 104
Chocolate
  Chocolate Avocado
    Pudding, 120
  Chocolate Coconut
    "Oatmeal," 48
  Chocolate Peanut
    Butter Cups, 129
  Chocolate Sea Salt
    Almonds, 116
  Cookie Dough, 123
  Cookies and Cream
    Parfait, 118
  Fat Hot Chocolate, 34–35
  French Vanilla Ice Cream
    with Hot Fudge, 122
  "Frosty" Chocolate
    Shake, 121
  Fudge Brownies, 127
  Mint Chocolate Fat
    Bombs, 132
  No-Bake Coconut
    Cookies, 124
  Walnut Zucchini Bread, 128
  Zucchini Chocolate
    Muffins, 46
Classic Buttermilk Syrup, 147
Classic Club Salad, 57
Classic Creamy Coleslaw, 54
Cloud Bread, 144

Coconut
  Chocolate Coconut
    "Oatmeal," 48
  Coconut Flaxseed Waffles, 47
  No-Bake Coconut
    Cookies, 124
  Superfood Granola, 38
Coconut milk
  Chocolate Avocado
    Pudding, 120
  Chocolate Coconut
    "Oatmeal," 48
  Coconut Iced Coffee, 142
  Creamy Snickerdoodle
    Shake, 37
  Kale Refresher Smoothie, 32
  Spirulina Smoothie, 33
  Tofu Green Bean
    Casserole, 100
  Vegan Coconut Curry, 103
Coffee
  Coconut Iced Coffee, 142
  Fat Coffee, 34
  Matcha Coffee, 36
Cookie Dough, 123
Cookies and Cream
  Parfait, 118
Cottage Cheese Salad,
  Greek, 56
Cream cheese
  Broccoli and Cauliflower
    Rice Casserole, 105
  Cheesy Cauliflower Mac
    'n' Cheese, 112
  Cheesy Dill Fat Bombs, 92
  Cloud Bread, 144
  Cream Cheese Pumpkin
    Muffins, 49
  Creamed Spinach
    with Eggs, 39
  Creamy Spinach Dip, 78
  "Everything but the Bagel"
    Fat Bombs, 91
  Fathead Crackers, 145
  Keto Cheesecake, 133–134

Mediterranean Cucumber
Bites, 76
Queso Blanco Dip, 146
Slow Cooker Broccoli
Cheese Soup, 67
Strawberry Cheesecake
Fat Bombs, 135
Three-Cheese Stuffed
Mushrooms, 88
Cream Cheese Pumpkin
Muffins, 49
Creamed Cauliflower Soup, 69
Creamed Spinach with Eggs, 39
Creamy Snickerdoodle
Shake, 37
Creamy Spinach Dip, 78
Creamy Stuffed Peppers, 101
Cucumbers
Classic Club Salad, 57
Greek Cottage Cheese
Salad, 56
Hemp Cobb Salad, 58
Kale Refresher Smoothie, 32
Loaded Bell Pepper
Sandwich, 65
Mediterranean Cucumber
Bites, 76
Mediterranean Salad, 59
Spinach Avocado Salad, 55
Curried Egg Salad, 52

D

Dairy-free
Almond Butter Pancakes, 45
Avocado Egg Salad, 53
Avocado Lime Dressing, 140
Broccoli Stir-Fry, 98
Cauliflower Fried Rice, 106
Chocolate Avocado
Pudding, 120
Chocolate Coconut
"Oatmeal," 48
Chocolate Peanut
Butter Cups, 129
Classic Creamy Coleslaw, 54

Creamy Snickerdoodle
Shake, 37
Curried Egg Salad, 52
Easy Keto Bread, 143
Flaxseed Chips and
Guacamole, 80
Green Goddess
Buddha Bowl, 96
Kale and Cashew Stir-Fry, 99
Kale Refresher Smoothie, 32
Lemon Bars, 125
Matcha Coffee, 36
Mint Chocolate Fat
Bombs, 132
No-Fail Deviled Eggs, 90
Peanut Butter Cookies, 126
Roasted Cauliflower
Hummus, 77
Roasted Cauliflower
Lettuce Cups, 62
Savory Party Mix, 89
Spinach Avocado
Salad, 55
Spirulina Smoothie, 33
Superfood Granola, 38
Thai Noodle Salad, 61
Vegan Coconut Curry, 103
Zucchini Chocolate
Muffins, 46
Desserts
Chocolate Avocado
Pudding, 120
Chocolate Peanut
Butter Cups, 129
Chocolate Sea Salt
Almonds, 116
Cookie Dough, 123
Cookies and Cream
Parfait, 118
French Vanilla Ice Cream
with Hot Fudge, 122
"Frosty" Chocolate
Shake, 121
Fudge Brownies, 127
Keto Cheesecake, 133–134

Keto-Friendly Key Lime
Pie, 130–131
Lemon Bars, 125
Mint Chocolate Fat
Bombs, 132
No-Bake Coconut
Cookies, 124
Peanut Butter Cookies, 126
Pecan Pie Pudding, 119
Salted Caramel Cashew
Brittle, 117
Strawberry Cheesecake
Fat Bombs, 135
Walnut Zucchini Bread, 128
Dining out, 14–15
Dips and spreads
Creamy Spinach Dip, 78
Flaxseed Chips and
Guacamole, 80
Quick and Easy
Ranch Dip, 141
Roasted Cauliflower
Hummus, 77

E

Easy Keto Bread, 143
Egg-free
Almond Butter Pancakes, 45
Avocado and Asparagus
Salad, 60
Avocado Lime Dressing, 140
Avocado Pesto Panini, 64
Avocado Pesto Zoodles, 138
Broccoli and Cauliflower
Rice Casserole, 105
Broccoli Stir-Fry, 98
Caprese Stuffed
Avocados, 82
Cauliflower Rice, 139
Cheesy Cauliflower Mac
'n' Cheese, 112
Cheesy Dill Fat Bombs, 92
Chiles Rellenos, 104
Chocolate Avocado
Pudding, 120

Egg-free (*continued*)

Chocolate Coconut "Oatmeal," 48

Chocolate Peanut Butter Cups, 129

Chocolate Sea Salt Almonds, 116

Classic Buttermilk Syrup, 147

Classic Creamy Coleslaw, 54

Coconut Iced Coffee, 142

Cookie Dough, 123

Cookies and Cream Parfait, 118

Creamed Cauliflower Soup, 69

Creamy Snickerdoodle Shake, 37

Creamy Spinach Dip, 78

"Everything but the Bage" Fat Bombs, 91

Fakeachini Alfredo, 111

Fat Chai, 35

Fat Coffee, 34

Fat Hot Chocolate, 34–35

Flaxseed Chips and Guacamole, 80

French Vanilla Ice Cream with Hot Fudge, 122

"Frosty" Chocolate Shake, 121

Greek Cottage Cheese Salad, 56

Green Goddess Buddha Bowl, 96

Instant Pot French Onion Soup, 68

Kale and Cashew Stir-Fry, 99

Kale Refresher Smoothie, 32

Loaded Bell Pepper Sandwich, 65

Matcha Coffee, 36

Mediterranean Cucumber Bites, 76

Mediterranean Salad, 59

Mexican Zucchini Hash, 107

Mint Chocolate Fat Bombs, 132

No-Bake Coconut Cookies, 124

Parmesan Zucchini Chips, 79

Pecan Pie Pudding, 119

Portobello Mushroom Burger with Avocado, 70

Queso Blanco Dip, 146

Quick and Easy Ranch Dip, 141

Roasted Cauliflower Lettuce Cups, 62

Roasted Garlic Mushrooms, 75

Salted Caramel Cashew Brittle, 117

Savory Party Mix, 89

Slow Cooker Broccoli Cheese Soup, 67

Smoked Almonds, 74

Spaghetti Squash Bake, 109

Spirulina Smoothie, 33

Strawberry Cheesecake Fat Bombs, 135

Superfood Granola, 38

Taco Lettuce Cups, 63

Thai Noodle Salad, 61

Three-Cheese Stuffed Mushrooms, 88

Tofu Green Bean Casserole, 100

Vegan Coconut Curry, 103

Zucchini Pizza Boats, 102

Zucchini Sage Pasta, 97

Eggplant Lasagna, 108

Eggs

Avocado Egg Salad, 53

Broccoli Quiche, 44

Cauliflower Fried Rice, 106

Classic Club Salad, 57

Cloud Bread, 144

Creamed Spinach with Eggs, 39

Curried Egg Salad, 52

Easy Keto Bread, 143

Eggs Benedict with Five-Minute Hollandaise, 43

Hemp Cobb Salad, 58

Italian Vegetable Egg Bake, 42

Keto Cheesecake, 133–134

Lemon Bars, 125

Mexican Egg Casserole, 40–41

No-Fail Deviled Eggs, 90

Spinach Avocado Salad, 55

Equipment, 11

"Everything but the Bagel" Fat Bombs, 91

F

Fakeachini Alfredo, 111

Fat bombs

Cheesy Dill Fat Bombs, 92

"Everything but the Bagel" Fat Bombs, 91

Mint Chocolate Fat Bombs, 132

Strawberry Cheesecake Fat Bombs, 135

Fat Chai, 35

Fat Coffee, 34

Fathead Crackers, 145

Fat Hot Chocolate, 34–35

Fats, 3–4

Flaxseed Chips and Guacamole, 80

French Vanilla Ice Cream with Hot Fudge, 122

"Frosty" Chocolate Shake, 121

Fudge Brownies, 127

G

Gluten-free

Almond Butter Pancakes, 45

Avocado and Asparagus Salad, 60

Avocado Egg Salad, 53

Avocado Lime Dressing, 140

Avocado Pesto Panini, 64

Avocado Pesto Zoodles, 138

Broccoli and Cauliflower Rice Casserole, 105

Broccoli Quiche, 44

Caprese Stuffed Avocados, 82

Cauliflower Fried Rice, 106

Cauliflower Rice, 139

Cheesy Cauliflower Breadsticks, 83–84

Cheesy Cauliflower Mac 'n' Cheese, 112

Cheesy Crackers, 81

Cheesy Dill Fat Bombs, 92

Cheesy Spinach Bake, 110

Chiles Rellenos, 104

Chocolate Avocado Pudding, 120

Chocolate Coconut "Oatmeal," 48

Chocolate Peanut Butter Cups, 129

Chocolate Sea Salt Almonds, 116

Classic Buttermilk Syrup, 147

Classic Club Salad, 57

Cloud Bread, 144

Coconut Flaxseed Waffles, 47

Coconut Iced Coffee, 142

Cookie Dough, 123

Cream Cheese Pumpkin Muffins, 49

Creamed Cauliflower Soup, 69

Creamed Spinach with Eggs, 39

Creamy Snickerdoodle Shake, 37

Creamy Spinach Dip, 78

Creamy Stuffed Peppers, 101

Curried Egg Salad, 52

Easy Keto Bread, 143

Eggplant Lasagna, 108

Eggs Benedict with Five-Minute Hollandaise, 43

"Everything but the Bagel" Fat Bombs, 91

Fat Chai, 35

Fat Coffee, 34

Fathead Crackers, 145

Fat Hot Chocolate, 34–35

Flaxseed Chips and Guacamole, 80

French Vanilla Ice Cream with Hot Fudge, 122

"Frosty" Chocolate Shake, 121

Fudge Brownies, 127

Greek Cottage Cheese Salad, 56

Green Goddess Buddha Bowl, 96

Hemp Cobb Salad, 58

Herbed Mozzarella Sticks, 85

Instant Pot French Onion Soup, 68

Italian Vegetable Egg Bake, 42

Kale and Cashew Stir-Fry, 99

Kale Refresher Smoothie, 32

Keto Cheesecake, 133–134

Keto-Friendly Key Lime Pie, 130–131

Lemon Bars, 125

Loaded Bell Pepper Sandwich, 65

Margherita Pizza, 113

Matcha Coffee, 36

Mediterranean Cucumber Bites, 76

Mediterranean Salad, 59

Mexican Egg Casserole, 40–41

Mexican Zucchini Hash, 107

Mint Chocolate Fat Bombs, 132

No-Bake Coconut Cookies, 124

No-Fail Deviled Eggs, 90

Parmesan Zucchini Chips, 79

Peanut Butter Cookies, 126

Pecan Pie Pudding, 119

Portobello Mushroom Burger with Avocado, 70

Queso Blanco Dip, 146

Quick and Easy Ranch Dip, 141

Roasted Cauliflower Hummus, 77

Roasted Cauliflower Lettuce Cups, 62

Roasted Garlic Mushrooms, 75

Salted Caramel Cashew Brittle, 117

Savory Party Mix, 89

Slow Cooker Broccoli Cheese Soup, 67

Smoked Almonds, 74

Spaghetti Squash Bake, 109

Spinach Avocado Salad, 55

Spirulina Smoothie, 33

Strawberry Cheesecake Fat Bombs, 135

Superfood Granola, 38

Taco Lettuce Cups, 63

Thai Noodle Salad, 61

Three-Cheese Stuffed Mushrooms, 88

Tofu Green Bean Casserole, 100

Ultimate Grilled Cheese, 66

Vegan Coconut Curry, 103

Walnut Zucchini Bread, 128

Zucchini Chocolate Muffins, 46

Zucchini Fritters, 87

Zucchini Pizza Boats, 102

Zucchini Sage Pasta, 97

Greek Cottage Cheese Salad, 56

Green Bean Tofu Casserole, 100

Green Goddess Buddha
Bowl, 96
Grocery shopping, 12

H

Hemp Cobb Salad, 58
Herbed Mozzarella Sticks, 85

I

Instant Pot French
Onion Soup, 68
Intermittent fasting, 13
Italian Vegetable Egg
Bake, 42

K

Kale and Cashew Stir-Fry, 99
Kale Refresher Smoothie, 32
Keto-adaptation, 5, 26–28
Keto Cheesecake,
133–134
Keto flu, 12–13
Keto-Friendly Key Lime
Pie, 130–131
Ketogenic diet, 2–3.
See also Vegetarian
ketogenic diet
Ketones, 2–3, 5
Ketosis, 2–3, 5

L

Lemon Bars, 125
Lettuce
Avocado and Asparagus
Salad, 60
Classic Club Salad, 57
Curried Egg Salad, 52
Loaded Bell Pepper
Sandwich, 65
Mediterranean Salad, 59
Roasted Cauliflower
Lettuce Cups, 62
Taco Lettuce Cups, 63
Limes
Avocado Lime Dressing, 140

Keto-Friendly Key Lime
Pie, 130–131
Loaded Bell Pepper
Sandwich, 65

M

Macronutrients, 3–4
Margherita Pizza, 113
Matcha Coffee, 36
Meal plans, 17
week 1, 18–21
week 2, 22–25
Meal prepping, 14
Meatless crumbles
Taco Lettuce Cups, 63
Mediterranean Cucumber
Bites, 76
Mediterranean Salad, 59
Mexican Egg Casserole, 40–41
Mexican Zucchini Hash, 107
Mint Chocolate Fat Bombs, 132
Muffins
Cream Cheese Pumpkin
Muffins, 49
Zucchini Chocolate
Muffins, 46
Mushrooms
Chiles Rellenos, 104
Mexican Zucchini Hash, 107
Portobello Mushroom
Burger with Avocado, 70
Roasted Garlic
Mushrooms, 75
Taco Lettuce Cups, 63
Three-Cheese Stuffed
Mushrooms, 88

N

Net carbs, 3
Neurological inflammation, 2–3
No-Bake Coconut Cookies, 124
No-Fail Deviled Eggs, 90
Noodle Salad, Thai, 61
Nut butters. *See also*
Peanut butter

Almond Butter Pancakes, 45
Chocolate Coconut
"Oatmeal," 48
Green Goddess
Buddha Bowl, 96
Matcha Coffee, 36
Salted Caramel Cashew
Brittle, 117
Thai Noodle Salad, 61
Nut-free
Avocado and Asparagus
Salad, 60
Avocado Egg Salad, 53
Avocado Lime Dressing, 140
Broccoli and Cauliflower
Rice Casserole, 105
Broccoli Quiche, 44
Broccoli Stir-Fry, 98
Cauliflower Fried Rice, 106
Cauliflower Rice, 139
Cheesy Cauliflower
Breadsticks, 83–84
Cheesy Cauliflower Mac
'n' Cheese, 112
Cheesy Dill Fat Bombs, 92
Cheesy Spinach Bake, 110
Chiles Rellenos, 104
Classic Buttermilk Syrup, 147
Classic Club Salad, 57
Classic Creamy Coleslaw, 54
Cloud Bread, 144
Coconut Flaxseed Waffles, 47
Coconut Iced Coffee, 142
Cookies and Cream
Parfait, 118
Creamed Cauliflower
Soup, 69
Creamy Spinach Dip, 78
Creamy Stuffed Peppers, 101
Eggplant Lasagna, 108
Eggs Benedict with Five-
Minute Hollandaise, 43
"Everything but the Bagel"
Fat Bombs, 91
Fakeachini Alfredo, 111

Fat Coffee, 34
Flaxseed Chips and
    Guacamole, 80
Greek Cottage Cheese
    Salad, 56
Hemp Cobb Salad, 58
Instant Pot French
    Onion Soup, 68
Italian Vegetable
    Egg Bake, 42
Loaded Bell Pepper
    Sandwich, 65
Margherita Pizza, 113
Mediterranean Cucumber
    Bites, 76
Mediterranean Salad, 59
Mexican Zucchini Hash, 107
No-Fail Deviled Eggs, 90
Parmesan Zucchini
    Chips, 79
Portobello Mushroom
    Burger with Avocado, 70
Queso Blanco Dip, 146
Quick and Easy
    Ranch Dip, 141
Roasted Cauliflower
    Hummus, 77
Roasted Garlic
    Mushrooms, 75
Slow Cooker Broccoli
    Cheese Soup, 67
Spaghetti Squash Bake, 109
Spinach Avocado
    Salad, 55
Strawberry Cheesecake
    Fat Bombs, 135
Three-Cheese Stuffed
    Mushrooms, 88
Tofu Green Bean
    Casserole, 100
Zucchini Chocolate
    Muffins, 46
Zucchini Pizza Boats, 102
Zucchini Sage Pasta, 97
Nutritional ketosis, 2–3, 5

Nuts
    Chocolate Sea Salt
        Almonds, 116
    Curried Egg Salad, 52
    Kale and Cashew
        Stir-Fry, 99
    Pecan Pie Pudding, 119
    Roasted Cauliflower
        Lettuce Cups, 62
    Salted Caramel Cashew
        Brittle, 117
    Savory Party Mix, 89
    Smoked Almonds, 74
    Superfood Granola, 38
    Thai Noodle Salad, 61
    Vegan Coconut Curry, 103
    Walnut Zucchini Bread, 128

O
Olives
    Baked Olives, 86
    Italian Vegetable
        Egg Bake, 42
    Mediterranean Cucumber
        Bites, 76
    Mediterranean Salad, 59
Onions
    Instant Pot French
        Onion Soup, 68

P
Parmesan Zucchini Chips, 79
Peanut butter
    Chocolate Peanut
        Butter Cups, 129
    No-Bake Coconut
        Cookies, 124
    Peanut Butter Cookies, 126
Pecan Pie Pudding, 119
Peppers. See Bell peppers
Pesto
    Avocado Pesto Panini, 64
    Avocado Pesto Zoodles, 138
    Caprese Stuffed
        Avocados, 82

Poblano chiles
    Chiles Rellenos, 104
Portobello Mushroom Burger
    with Avocado, 70
Protein, 3–4
Pumpkin Cream Cheese
    Muffins, 49

Q
Queso Blanco Dip, 146
Quick and Easy Ranch Dip, 141

R
Radishes
    Avocado Egg Salad, 53
Ricotta cheese
    Creamy Stuffed Peppers, 101
    Eggplant Lasagna, 108
    Zucchini Pizza Boats, 102
Roasted Cauliflower
    Hummus, 77
Roasted Cauliflower
    Lettuce Cups, 62
Roasted Garlic Mushrooms, 75

S
Salads
    Avocado and Asparagus
        Salad, 60
    Avocado Egg Salad, 53
    Classic Club Salad, 57
    Classic Creamy Coleslaw, 54
    Curried Egg Salad, 52
    Greek Cottage Cheese
        Salad, 56
    Hemp Cobb Salad, 58
    Mediterranean Salad, 59
    Roasted Cauliflower
        Lettuce Cups, 62
    Spinach Avocado Salad, 55
    Taco Lettuce Cups, 63
    Thai Noodle Salad, 61
Salt, 13
Salted Caramel Cashew
    Brittle, 117

Sandwiches
    Avocado Pesto Panini, 64
    Loaded Bell Pepper
        Sandwich, 65
    Portobello Mushroom
        Burger with Avocado, 70
    Ultimate Grilled Cheese, 66
Savory Party Mix, 89
Seitan
    Broccoli Stir-Fry, 98
    Classic Creamy Coleslaw, 54
    Fakeachini Alfredo, 111
    Slow Cooker Broccoli
        Cheese Soup, 67
Smoked Almonds, 74
Smoothies
    Creamy Snickerdoodle
        Shake, 37
    "Frosty" Chocolate
        Shake, 121
    Kale Refresher Smoothie, 32
    Spirulina Smoothie, 33
Soups
    Creamed Cauliflower
        Soup, 69
    Instant Pot French
        Onion Soup, 68
    Slow Cooker Broccoli
        Cheese Soup, 67
Spaghetti Squash Bake, 109
Spinach
    Broccoli Stir-Fry, 98
    Cheesy Spinach Bake, 110
    Chiles Rellenos, 104
    Creamed Spinach
        with Eggs, 39
    Creamy Spinach Dip, 78
    Creamy Stuffed Peppers, 101
    Green Goddess
        Buddha Bowl, 96
    Hemp Cobb Salad, 58
    Italian Vegetable
        Egg Bake, 42
    Mexican Egg
        Casserole, 40–41

Spinach Avocado Salad, 55
Zucchini Pizza Boats, 102
Zucchini Sage Pasta, 97
Spinach Avocado Salad, 55
Spirulina Smoothie, 33
Sprouts
    Portobello Mushroom
        Burger with Avocado, 70
Squash. See also Zucchini
    Fakeachini Alfredo, 111
    Spaghetti Squash
        Bake, 109
Strawberry Cheesecake
    Fat Bombs, 135
Sugar alcohols, 3
Superfood Granola, 38
Support networks, 15

T
Taco Lettuce Cups, 63
Tea
    Fat Chai, 35
    Matcha Coffee, 36
Thai Noodle Salad, 61
Three-Cheese Stuffed
    Mushrooms, 88
Tofu
    Tofu Green Bean
        Casserole, 100
    Zucchini Sage Pasta, 97
Tomatoes
    Avocado and Asparagus
        Salad, 60
    Caprese Stuffed
        Avocados, 82
    Classic Club Salad, 57
    Eggplant Lasagna, 108
    Greek Cottage Cheese
        Salad, 56
    Hemp Cobb Salad, 58
    Mediterranean Salad, 59
    Spinach Avocado Salad, 55
    Vegan Coconut Curry, 103
Tools, 11
Total carbs, 3

U
Ultimate Grilled Cheese, 66

V
Vegan Coconut Curry, 103
Vegetables. See also specific
    Kale and Cashew Stir-Fry, 99
Vegetarian ketogenic
        diet, 4–5
    foods to enjoy and avoid, 8–9
    meal plans, 18–25
    special ingredients, 10–11
    substitutions, 9–10
    tips, 12–15

W
Walnut Zucchini Bread, 128
Weight loss, 3

Y
Yogurt
    Broccoli Quiche, 44
    Cookies and Cream
        Parfait, 118
    Pecan Pie Pudding, 119
    Portobello Mushroom
        Burger with Avocado, 70
    Quick and Easy
        Ranch Dip, 141

Z
Zucchini
    Avocado Pesto Zoodles, 138
    Cheesy Spinach Bake, 110
    Mexican Zucchini Hash, 107
    Parmesan Zucchini
        Chips, 79
    Vegan Coconut Curry, 103
    Walnut Zucchini Bread, 128
    Zucchini Chocolate
        Muffins, 46
    Zucchini Fritters, 87
    Zucchini Pizza Boats, 102
    Zucchini Sage Pasta, 97

ACKNOWLEDGMENTS

I would like to thank my publisher, Callisto Media, for allowing me to write this book, as well as my editor, Justin Hartung, whose passion for the project was unwavering. I would also like to thank my husband, Ryan, and my children for their patience during the time it took me to complete this book.

ABOUT THE AUTHOR

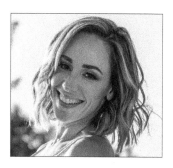

Lisa Danielson, aka Veggie Lisa, is a wife of 18 years and a mother of four children ranging in age from 6 to 15 years old. At one point in her life, Lisa weighed 200 pounds. After tweaking her diet to include more plant-based protein sources, she was able to lose almost 60 pounds. As a lifelong vegetarian, she has a passion for vegetables and loves teaching others how delicious they can be. She graduated from Brigham Young University with a degree in dance education; she is an ISSA Fitness Nutrition Specialist, Certified Personal Trainer, and a Corrective Exercise Specialist; and she teaches HIGH Fitness. She is the head nutritionist for a major protein supplement company and also helps her personal clients reach their weight-loss goals.

CPSIA information can be obtained
at www.ICGtesting.com
Printed in the USA
JSHW011908280122
22324JS00005B/5